T0348398

Update on Diagnosis and Treatment of Brain Tumors in Dogs and Cats

Editor

HELENA RYLANDER

VETERINARY CLINICS OF NORTH AMERICA: SMALL ANIMAL PRACTICE

www.vetsmall.theclinics.com

January 2025 • Volume 55 • Number 1

ELSEVIER

1600 John F. Kennedy Boulevard • Suite 1800 • Philadelphia, Pennsylvania, 19103-2899
http://www.vetsmall.theclinics.com

**VETERINARY CLINICS OF NORTH AMERICA: SMALL ANIMAL PRACTICE Volume 55, Number 1
January 2025 ISSN 0195-5616, ISBN-13: 978-0-443-31472-8**

Editor: Stacy Eastman
Developmental Editor: Varun Gopal

Veterinary Clinics of North America: Small Animal Practice (ISSN 0195-5616) is published bimonthly by Elsevier Inc., 360
Park Avenue South, New York, NY 10010-1710. Months of issue are January, March, May, July, September, and
November. Business and Editorial Offices: 1600 John F. Kennedy Blvd., Ste. 1800, Philadelphia, PA 19103-2899.
Customer Service Office: 3251 Riverport Lane, Maryland Heights, MO 63043. Periodicals postage paid at New York,
NY and additional mailing offices. Subscription prices are $403.00 per year (domestic individuals), $100.00 per year (domestic students/residents), $518.00 per year (Canadian individuals), $560.00 per year (international individuals), $100.00
per year (Canadian students/residents), and $220.00 per year (international students/residents). For institutional access
pricing please contact Customer Service via the contact information below. To receive student/resident rate, orders must
be accompanied by name of affiliated institution, date of term, and the *signature* of program/residency coordinator on
institution letterhead. Orders will be billed at individual rate until proof of status is received. Foreign air speed delivery is
included in all *Clinics* subscription prices. All prices are subject to change without notice. Orders, claims, and journal in-
quiries: Please visit our Support Hub page https://service.elsevier.com for assistance.

Reprints. For copies of 100 or more of articles in this publication, please contact the Commercial Reprints Department,
Elsevier Inc., 360 Park Avenue South, New York, NY 10010-1710. Tel.: 212-633-3874; Fax: 212-633-3820; E-mail:
reprints@elsevier.com.

Veterinary Clinics of North America: Small Animal Practice is also published in Japanese by Inter Zoo Publishing Co.,
Ltd., Aoyama Crystal-Bldg 5F, 3-5-12 Kitaaoyama, Minato-ku, Tokyo 107-0061, Japan.

Veterinary Clinics of North America: Small Animal Practice is covered in *Current Contents/Agriculture, Biology and Envi-
ronmental Sciences, Science Citation Index, ASCA, MEDLINE/PubMed (Index Medicus), Excerpta Medica,* and *BIOSIS.*
Printed in the United States of America.

Contributors

EDITOR

HELENA RYLANDER, DVM
Diplomate of the American College of Veterinary Internal Medicine (Neurology); Clinical Professor, UW Madison, School of Veterinary Medicine, Madison, Wisconsin, USA

AUTHORS

SHEILA CARRERA-JUSTIZ, DVM
Diplomate of the American College of Veterinary Internal Medicine (Neurology); Clinical Associate Professor, Small Animal Clinical Sciences, College of Veterinary Medicine, University of Florida, Gainesville, Florida, USA

TRACY L. GIEGER, DVM
Clinical Professor, Department of Clinical Sciences, College of Veterinary Medicine, North Carolina State University, Raleigh, North Carolina, USA

NICK D. JEFFERY, BVSc, PhD, MSc, FRCVS
Diplomate European College of Veterinary Neurology; Diplomate European College of Veterinary Surgery; Professor, Neurology & Neurosurgery, Department of Small Animal Clinical Sciences, College of Veterinary Medicine and Biomedical Sciences, Texas A&M University, College Station, Texas, USA

MICHAEL S. KENT, DVM, MAS
Diplomate of the American College of Veterinary Internal Medicine (MO), Diplomate of the American College of Veterinary Radiology (RO), Diplomate, European College of Veterinary Diagnostic Imaging (RO); Professor, Department of Surgical and Radiological Sciences, School of Veterinary Medicine, University of California Davis, Davis, California, USA

SIMON T. KORNBERG, BVSc
Diplomate of the American College of Veterinary Internal Medicine (Neurology); Veterinary Neurologist, Southeast Veterinary Neurology, Miami, Florida, USA

ALISON M. LEE, DVM, MS
Diplomate of the American College of Veterinary Radiology; Associate Professor and Section Chief, Department of Clinical Science, College of Veterinary Medicine, Mississippi State University, Mississippi State, Mississippi, USA

SAMANTHA LOEBER, DVM
Diplomate of the American College of Veterinary Radiology, Diplomate of the American College of Veteirnary Imaging-Equine Diagnostic Imaging; Diplomate of the American College of Veterinary Radiology-Equine Diagnostic Imaging; Clinical Assistant Professor of Diagnostic Imaging, Department of Surgical Sciences, University of Wisconsin-Madison, Madison, Wisconsin, USA

BJÖRN P. MEIJ, DVM, PhD
Diplomate of the European College of Veterinary Surgeons; Professor and Head, Small Animal Surgery, Department of Clinical Sciences, Faculty of Veterinary Medicine, Utrecht University, Utrecht, The Netherlands

MICHELLE L. MENDOZA, DVM
Resident, Department of Clinical Science, College of Veterinary Medicine, Mississippi State University, Mississippi State, Mississippi, USA

MATTHIAS ROSSEEL, DVM
Resident, William R. Pritchard Veterinary Medical Teaching Hospital, School of Veterinary Medicine, University of California Davis, Davis, California, USA

JOHN H. ROSSMEISL DVM, MS
Diplomate American College of Veterinary Internal Medicine (Small Animal Internal Medicine and Neurology); Dr. John H. Rossmeisl Dr and Mrs Dorothy Taylor Mahin Professor of Neurology and Neurosurgery, Veterinary and Comparative Neuro-oncology Laboratory, Department of Small Animal Clinical Sciences, Virginia-Maryland College of Veterinary Medicine, Virginia Tech, Blacksburg, Virginia, USA

KATHARINE RUSSELL, MVB
Resident, Southeast Veterinary Neurology, Miami, Florida, USA

ANDY SHORES, DVM, MS, PhD
Diplomate of the American College of Veterinary Internal Medicine (Neurology); Clinical Professor and Section Chief, Department of Clinical Science, College of Veterinary Medicine, Mississippi State University, Mississippi State, Mississippi, USA

LUCINDA L. VAN STEE, DVM
Diplomate of the European College of Veterinary Surgeons; Clinician, Small Animal Surgery, Department of Clinical Sciences, Faculty of Veterinary Medicine, Utrecht University, Utrecht, The Netherlands

Contents

> Meningiomas are the most common tumor type in the brain in dogs and cats, and survival times are much higher for cats than dogs. Glioma is much more common in the dog, and median survival time is poor without definitive therapy. No recommendations currently exist for treatment of glioma in dogs, and there is ongoing research as the dog is a valid spontaneous model for the human equivalent disease. Other intracranial tumor types like lymphoma and histiocytic sarcoma do occur, though at a much lower frequency.

> MRI plays an integral role in the diagnosis of brain tumors in dogs and cats. Optimized image acquisition protocols in addition to a systematic approach to brain tumor evaluation on MRI using imaging characteristic interpretation criteria may allow for enhanced lesion detection, accurate presumptive diagnoses, and formulation of a prioritized differential diagnosis list.

> Extensive descriptions of MRI characteristics of canine and feline brain tumors allow for relatively accurate lesion detection, discrimination, and presumptive diagnosis on MRI. Ambiguous and overlapping MRI features between brain lesion and tumor as well as tumor types is a limitation that necessitates histopathology for final diagnosis, which is often not available antemortem. Non-invasive advanced diagnostic imaging techniques continue to be developed to enhance sensitivity and specificity for brain tumor diagnosis on MRI in dogs and cats.

> Brain biopsy is essential for accurate diagnosis but is frequently avoided in veterinary medicine because of doubts about its safety, reliability, and clinical value. Data available from human and veterinary investigations suggest that such doubts are largely unwarranted. Many devices are available to guide minimally invasive biopsy but some can be costly to

purchase and use, which can be problematic in veterinary medicine. Nowadays, costs can be substantially reduced by using 3-dimensional-printed guides.

with wider availability of advanced imaging, together with more challenging cases. In this review, the current state of hypophysectomy is described with future challenges and opportunities.

Radiation therapy for the treatment of both functional and nonfunctional pituitary tumors for dogs and cats has been described in veterinary medicine with a recent shift in focus toward stereotactic techniques. While the technology required and normal tissue constraints for stereotactic procedures are more stringent, recent publications indicate that, while it helps alleviate clinical signs, the survival response may not be as durable as with conventionally fractionated radiation therapy in dogs, despite being seen in cats. Regardless of the protocol recommendation, potential benefit to the patient is excellent with manageable side effect profiles.

Brain tumors exert their clinical effects in a variety of ways. Mass effect, edema, seizures, and a vicious cycle of cause and effect are often the focus of therapeutic interventions employed to improve clinical signs and increase survival time. Obstructive hydrocephalus is a common sequela of certain types of brain tumors and is often the major driver of clinical signs seen in tumors arising within the ventricular system. This study outlines the application of ventriculoperitoneal shunting for obstructive hydrocephalus secondary to brain tumors as part of an overall management program to help increase patients' lifespan and quality of life.

 Video content accompanies this article at http://www.vetsmall. theclinics.com.

This study describes the essential components and the technique of intraoperative ultrasound (IOUS), including probe selection and techniques used to produce quality images. Case examples are given to illustrate the value and the accuracy of IOUS in intracranial surgery of companion animals. IOUS has proven an invaluable addition to intracranial surgery, especially in real-time localization of the mass, identifying borders between mass and normal cerebral tissue, and identifying vascular supply to the mass.

VETERINARY CLINICS OF NORTH AMERICA: SMALL ANIMAL PRACTICE

SERIES OF RELATED INTEREST

Veterinary Clinics: Exotic Animal Practice
https://www.vetexotic.theclinics.com/
Advances in Small Animal Care
https://www.advancesinsmallanimalcare.com/

THE CLINICS ARE NOW AVAILABLE ONLINE!
Access your subscription at:
www.theclinics.com

Preface

Update on Diagnosis and Treatment of Brain Tumors in Dogs and Cats

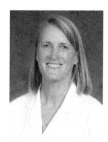

Helena Rylander, DVM
Editor

I am excited to present a new issue of *Veterinary Clinics of North America: Small Animal Practice* featuring the diagnosis and treatment of brain tumors in dogs and cats. When I have a patient with a brain lesion, I often think of Harvey Cushing, who at the beginning of the twentieth century with help of a thorough neurologic examination was able to localize the exact location of a lesion without the help of any diagnostic imaging or even an X ray. He performed over 2000 procedures, including brain surgeries, during his career, and by inventing new instruments, such as vascular clips to prevent hemorrhage, improving instruments and developing his surgical technique, the mortality for brain surgeries was reduced from 50% to 10%.

A lot has happened in this field since then with more eloquent techniques helping us come up with a more definitive diagnosis, or at least a shorter list of differential diagnoses for brain lesions seen on MRI. Since the last *Veterinary Clinics of North America: Small Animal Practice* issue featuring diseases of the brain, 14 years ago, things have continued to evolve in diagnostics, imaging, and treatment of brain tumors.

The first article by Dr Carrera-Justiz is a nice summary of the diagnosis and treatment of brain tumors. Dr Loeber discusses MRI in two articles, with the first talking about standard protocols and the second one describing more in detail MRI features of different brain tumors and new imaging techniques. Dr Jeffery discusses biopsy of brain tumor, something that is not done often enough. With any surgeries, complications can occur, and Dr Shores nicely describes them in his article. Radiation therapy is a field where things progress very rapidly, and Dr Geiger gives us a nice overview in her article. New treatments are being undertaken as part of many research protocols, and some may become available in the near future for our clinical patients, something that Dr Rossmeisl discusses. Dr Meij at the University in Utrecht was the pioneer in

Vet Clin Small Anim 55 (2025) ix–x
https://doi.org/10.1016/j.cvsm.2024.07.001
0195-5616/25/© 2024 Published by Elsevier Inc.

doing surgery for pituitary tumors in our patients, so it is very appropriate that he discusses this in his article. Radiation therapy for pituitary tumors has been studied vastly at UC Davis, and Dr Kent summarizes this treatment. We get an update on ventriculoperitoneal shunting by Dr Kornberg, and Dr Shores tells us about how intraoperative ultrasound can improve the surgical outcome in brain surgery.

I would like to thank the authors for taking the time to contribute to this issue. They are already very busy being clinicians, teachers, and researchers, and I am so thankful that they took the time to share their expertise on this topic.

Helena Rylander, DVM
UW Madison
School of Veterinary Medicine
2015 Linden Drive
Madison, WI 53706, USA

E-mail address:
Helena.rylander@wisc.edu

Introduction and Summary of Diagnosis and Treatment of Brain Tumors in Dogs and Cats

Sheila Carrera-Justiz, DVM*

KEYWORDS

- Brain tumor • Meningioma • Glioma • Intracranial histiocytic sarcoma

KEY POINTS

- In cats with intracranial meningioma, surgery alone can yield a survival time of 3 years.
- Survival time of dogs with intracranial neoplasia is improved with definitive therapy.
- Glioma can be difficult to definitively diagnose on imaging alone.
- To improve survival time in dogs with glioma, multimodal therapy is required.
- Central nervous system histiocytic sarcoma has a very poor prognosis.

INTRODUCTION

Brain tumors in dogs and cats are now a well-recognized phenomenon. Primary central nervous system (CNS) neoplasia in dogs is reported at 14.5 cases per 100,000 while in cats it is less common at about 3.5 per 100,000 cases.[1,2]

Despite intracranial surgery becoming more commonplace, it is not always an option, and a presumptive diagnosis is made based on imaging findings, which then guides both therapeutic and prognostic recommendations. An extensive body of literature is now available to help make an informed diagnosis based on imaging findings, and there is still more work to be done to improve this process.[3] The dog has been established as a model of human glioma, as its glioma is naturally occurring, and this recognition has allowed for advances in treatment of glioma in dogs and humans.[4–6]

Despite recent advances in canine and feline intracranial neoplasia, challenges will always exist and much remains to be discovered. Median survival time in dogs with palliatively treated brain tumors is generally poor at 69 days. Dogs with infratentorial tumors have a significantly shorter median survival time than dogs with supratentorial tumors at 28 versus 178 days, respectively.[7] This information is relatively unknown for cats, though can likely be extrapolated from dogs.

Small Animal Clinical Sciences, College of Veterinary Medicine, University of Florida, PO Box 100126, Gainesville, FL 32610, USA
* 10283 Southwest 36th Place, Gainesville, FL 32608.
E-mail address: Carrerajustiz.s@ufl.edu

Vet Clin Small Anim 55 (2025) 1–9
https://doi.org/10.1016/j.cvsm.2024.07.002
0195-5616/25/© 2024 Elsevier Inc. All rights reserved, including those for text and data mining, AI training, and similar technologies.

MENINGIOMA

Meningioma is the most common intracranial tumor type identified in dogs and cats, though the presentation and behavior are different in each species. It has recently been determined that cats have larger meningioma than dogs, which may reflect the biological differences of the tumor in the different species.[8]

Canine Meningioma

The most common presenting complaint of dogs with meningioma is seizures.[8] Rostrotentorial meningiomas have a median survival time of 422 days with surgery alone, though presence of a midline shift and ventricular compression can have a negative effect on survival time.[9] Median survival time of dogs that had a transfrontal approach was 184 days while dogs that had a rostrotentorial approach had a median survival time of 646 days, which may reflect the more limited exposure associated with the former compared to the latter.[10] As was suggested by prior studies, surgical resection of canine meningiomas performed with a surgical aspirator can increase median survival times to more than 2 years with no adjunctive treatment.[11]

Feline Meningioma

Meningioma is the most common primary CNS neoplasm in cats representing 85% of primary brain neoplasms.[2] Meningioma is a disease of middle-aged to geriatric cats with the most common presenting complaint being behavior changes.[8] Interestingly, up to 20% of meningiomas in cats can be clinically silent and incidental, likely a reflection of the benign and slow growing nature of these tumors. Cats tend to have larger tumors than dogs and it is common to find foraminal herniation.[8] Calvarial hyperostosis is a common finding. The mechanism of this is not well understood, but a recent study showed that tumor invasion into abnormal bone occurred in almost half of the cats studied.[12] Surgical resection is the treatment of choice due to the benign and slow-growing nature of feline meningiomas. The most recent study looking at survival after surgical resection showed that cats have a median survival time of about 3 years with no additional intervention such as chemotherapy or radiation therapy.[13]

GLIOMA

Glioma continues to be a common brain tumor diagnosis in the dog, especially brachycephalic dogs. A large proportion of dogs present with an acute onset of seizures and almost half present with cluster seizures or status epilepticus as the initial onset.[14] Glioma can be challenging to distinguish from other neurologic lesions, and they can be especially difficult to further characterize purely based on imaging.[15,16] MRI findings correlate better with tumor grade than tumor type, with contrast enhancement, gradient echo signal voids, and T2W-heterogeneity all increasing with increasing grade.[15] The reported median survival time for dogs with glioma treated palliatively ranges from 26 to 60 days.[14,17,18,] Canine glioma has recently been documented to disseminate within the CNS via drop metastasis. These metastases were all noted to be downstream, in the direction of cerebrospinal fluid (CSF) flow, and the metastasis may have very different imaging characteristics to the parent tumor.[19]

Feline glioma is a less well-described condition. One retrospective study describes the histologic findings in 13 cases from 2 institutions over 16 years, supporting the rarity of this condition in cats.[20] Glioma is the third or fourth most common primary CNS neoplasm of cats and makes up about 12% of primary brain neoplasms. In cats, astrocytoma is the most common glial tumor, followed by ependymoma, oligodendroglioma, and then other rare glioma subtypes.[20]

Definitive Treatment

Surgical resection alone for treatment of glioma has the same median survival time as with palliative therapy, suggesting that definitive treatment of glioma requires multimodal therapy.[7,9] In dogs with glioma undergoing surgery with or without adjunctive treatment, preoperative tumor size has no impact on outcome or survival.[9,21] However, tumor grade, which requires biopsy for definitive diagnosis, is predictive of outcome, with median survival times for low-grade and high-grade tumors being 727 and 174 days, respectively, in dogs receiving combination therapy.[21]

LYMPHOMA

CNS lymphoma as part of multicentric lymphoma is the second most common intracranial tumor in cats, though primary CNS lymphoma is rare, and it is the most common neoplasm affecting the spinal cord of cats.[2,22] In the cat, intracranial lymphoma often causes either a diffuse parenchymal infiltration or a subependymal infiltration.[22] Despite lymphoma being a very common nervous system neoplasia in cats, MRI features are extremely varied in both cats and dogs, which can make diagnosis a challenge.[23]

In the dog, primary nervous system lymphoma is much less frequent than secondary lymphoma, with a slightly higher preponderance of B-cell over T-cell lymphoma subtypes.[24] CNS lymphoma is notoriously difficult to diagnose due to the varied presentation and diagnostic imaging findings. An ante-mortem diagnosis is ideally made with a combination of cytology of CSF and MRI findings. Historically, survival time of dogs with CNS lymphoma with any treatment was less than 3 months. Recent literature has shown a median survival time in dogs with CNS lymphoma of 171 days (range 1–1942 days), with dogs receiving treatment having longer survival times than those not receiving any treatment.[25] Histologic findings indicate that dogs with nervous system lymphoma and a CSF pleocytosis above 64 cells/μL tend to have marked meningeal and periventricular infiltration, characteristic of diffuse large B-cell lymphoma.[24]

Nervous system lymphoma is notorious for its varied and unpredictable clinical presentation and imaging findings. A recent report described a novel presentation of 6 animals (5 dogs and 1 cat) with intracranial lymphoma and choroid plexus involvement.[26] Intravascular lymphoma, which has historically been a post-mortem diagnosis, has recently been shown to have unique characteristics on MRI. Evidence of ischemic lesions in diffusion-weighted imaging, as well as susceptibility artifacts on gradient recalled echo images, correlate with the histopathological findings of dilated vessels plugged by neoplastic cells.[27] The combination of ischemic and hemorrhagic lesions on imaging now should include intravascular lymphoma as a potential cause.

HISTIOCYTIC SARCOMA

Histiocytic sarcoma is a round cell neoplasia that can affect the nervous system as part of disseminated disease or it can be limited to the nervous system. Retrievers and Pembroke Welsh Corgies seem to be overrepresented in this disease, as are Bernese Mountain Dogs, Rottweilers, and Shetland Sheepdogs. The survival time is extremely poor at 3 to 4 days. In the brain, histiocytic sarcoma mostly causes extra-axial masses with meningeal enhancement that may be distant from the mass. CSF pleocytosis is useful in the diagnosis of histiocytic sarcoma. Marked pleocytosis is seen mostly with primary and not disseminated disease, and neoplastic cells may be identified cytologically. Similar to other neoplasia in the CNS, dogs that underwent definitive treatment survived longer than those with palliative treatment.[28,29]

CURRENT EVIDENCE

In veterinary medicine, there is little evidence that one treatment modality is better than another for treatment of intracranial neoplasia. Evidence does show that survival for dogs with intracranial neoplasia is longer with some form of definitive treatment.[18] Palliative treatment of intracranial neoplasia has traditionally consisted of corticosteroid therapy to reduce peritumoral edema and anticonvulsant therapy, as needed to control seizures. Definitive treatment can include surgery, chemotherapy, radiation therapy, or any combination thereof.

Surgery

Short-term survival after intracranial surgery in dogs is excellent and most complications are not life threatening, suggesting that technical skills, patient selection, and protocols are good.[30,31] Thirteen percent of dogs that underwent intracranial surgery for a rostrotentorial lesion had early postoperative seizures, and those dogs had prolonged hospitalization, more complications, and shorter survival time than dogs without postoperative seizures.[32] It should be noted that in the study by Forward and colleagues, the majority of patients were diagnosed with meningioma or non-neoplastic disease while the study by Parker and colleagues included a variety of neoplasias.

Chemotherapy

A study evaluating the utility of oral lomustine in dogs with presumptive intracranial glioma showed that median survival time can be significantly extended from 35 to 138 days.[18] However, a meta analysis of the veterinary literature did not find support for the use of lomustine in the treatment of brain tumors.[33] Lomustine and other chemotherapeutics are not without side effects, and lomustine-related side effects are common.

Radiotherapy

Radiation therapy is a viable treatment option in many cases of intracranial neoplasia. It has been shown to be a useful modality in cats, helping to relieve clinical signs and improve local tumor control for a variety of neoplastic processes.[34] Three-dimensional conformal radiation therapy has been shown to induce a longer survival time than glucocorticoids alone in dogs with infratentorial brain tumors, extending median survival time from 89 to 756 days.[35] Stereotactic radiotherapy (SRT) is also increasing in use in veterinary medicine. In a study of 11 dogs with intraventricular masses that received SRT, the overall median survival time from the first SRT treatment was almost 17 months, with a range of 24 to 1960 days. Dogs with moderate to marked ventriculomegaly and carcinoma had shorter survival times than those without.[36] Both stereotactic radiosurgery and SRTs have been shown to reduce tumor volume and perfusion in multiple tumor types including suspected and definitively diagnosed meningioma, pituitary masses, and glioma.[37]

Combination Therapy

A study combining surgical resection with metronomic chlorambucil for treatment of canine glioma showed the potential for prolonged seizure control as well as a median overall survival time of 257 days.[38] Dogs undergoing surgical resection of glioma followed by temozolamide therapy had a median survival time of 240 days.[39] These studies showed a marked improvement in median survival time over the 60 days reported with no treatment, supporting the idea that glioma therapy requires a multipronged approach.

EMERGING THERAPIES/EMERGING TREATMENT

Traditional surgical approaches to the cranial vault include transfrontal, rostrotentorial, caudotentorial or occipital, and transsphenoidal techniques. Many of these approaches can be combined to allow for appropriate access to the underlying nervous structures. A novel surgical approach was recently described that allows access to lesions in the olfactory bulb and frontal lobe caudomedial to the orbit. The transorbital craniectomy is performed and spares the globe while allowing improved access to disease medial to the orbital aspect of the temporal bone.[40] Techniques are also developing to improve intraoperative identification of neoplastic versus normal tissue.[41]

CHALLENGES

Definitive diagnosis of any brain mass still requires histopathology, though some tumors have more typical imaging characteristics than others. Most meningiomas in dogs and cats have a classic appearance and are reliably diagnosed on MRI, though atypical meningiomas pose a diagnostic challenge. Glioma is much more challenging to diagnose as there are many glioma mimics, and MRI characteristics correlate more to tumor grade than type.[15,16] Proton MR spectroscopy has the capacity to distinguish inflammatory from neoplastic lesions, though this technique is not yet widespread.[42,43]

CURRENT CONTROVERSIES

Ideal treatment recommendations for intracranial neoplasia in the dog and cat do not currently exist. Considering the prolonged survival time of cats after surgical resection of an intracranial meningioma with no adjunctive therapy, surgery alone seems to be a good recommendation for the cat.[13] Historically, a recommendation of surgical resection of an intracranial meningioma in the dog, followed by radiation therapy was accepted as best practice, and both modalities are frequently offered as sole treatment options. A recent study reviewed a large number of cases that underwent surgical resection of a meningioma followed by various adjunctive treatments; no clear benefit on survival time was found with any adjunctive treatment.[10] Much debate persists as to whether surgery or radiation therapy is a better treatment recommendation for dogs with meningioma. Further studies with standardized treatment protocols are required to identify the ideal treatment for canine meningioma.

FUTURE CONSIDERATIONS

Biopsy of intracranial lesions is becoming more common in dogs, and it is generally a well-tolerated procedure.[44] It is crucial for the continued improvement in diagnosis and treatment of intracranial neoplasia that a definitive diagnosis is made, be this through biopsy, surgical resection, or necropsy. Novel imaging techniques are being studied to help definitively diagnose neoplasia in a non-invasive manner, and imaging findings must be correlated to histopathology.[42,43,45,46]

A consensus document has been produced that describes recommendations for MRI protocols for multicenter canine brain tumor clinical trials. Recommendations include precontrast and postcontrast 3 dimensional T1-weighted images, T2-weighted turbo spin echo in all 3 planes, T2*-weighted gradient recalled echo, T2-weighted fluid attenuated inversion recovery, and diffusion weighted imaging/diffusion tensor imaging in the transverse plane. Consistency in imaging protocols across institutions would reduce variation in large, multi-institutional studies and would allow for reliable translation of imaging data to human clinical trials.[47]

Considering the poor long-term outcome in humans with malignant glioma and the evidence for dogs as a spontaneous model for human glioma, much research is focused on glioma therapy. Irreversible electroporation, a minimally invasive, nonthermal treatment for solid tumors, has been shown to be effective for canine glioma.[48] Glioma is particularly difficult to treat due to being immunologically cold, and many groups are working on how to activate an immune response against the tumor. Much research is focusing on various immunotherapeutic routes, including vaccines, immune checkpoint inhibition, and nanoparticles as a vehicle for therapeutic payload.[49–54]

SUMMARY

Novel techniques for non-invasive identification of intracranial neoplasia are being developed and put into practice. Easier and more reliable identification of tumor types will allow for better treatment recommendations and will propel research in a forward direction. Studies evaluating new therapeutic modalities and combination therapies for glioma are showing improved outcomes and prolonged survival times.

DISCLOSURE

The author has nothing to disclose.

REFERENCES

1. Miller AD, Miller CR, Rossmeisl JH. Canine primary intracranial cancer: a clinicopathologic and comparative review of glioma, meningioma, and choroid plexus tumors. Front in Onc 2019;9:1151.
2. Rissi DR. A review of primary central nervous system neoplasms of cats. Vet Path 2023;60(3):294–307.
3. Bentley RT. Magnetic resonance imaging diagnosis of brain tumors in dogs. Vet J 2015;205:204–16.
4. Hicks WH, Bird CE, Pernik MN, et al. Large animal models of glioma: current status and future prospects. Anticancer Res 2021;41:5343–53.
5. Hubbard ME, Arnold S, Zahid AB, et al. Naturally occurring canine glioma as a model for novel therapeutics. Cancer Invest 2018;36(8):415–23.
6. LeBlanc A. A report from the NCI comparative brain tumor consortium (CBTC) glioma pathology board: a revised diagnostic classification in support of validation of the canine glioma patient as a model for humans. Vet Path 2019;56(4):642–3.
7. Rossmeisl JH, Jones JC, Zimmerman KL, et al. Survival time following hospital discharge in dogs with palliatively treated primary brain tumors. J Am Vet Med Assoc 2013;242:193–8.
8. Minato S, Cherubini GB, Della Santa D, et al. Incidence and type of brain herniation associated with intracranial meningioma in dogs and cats. J Vet Med Sci 2021;83(2):267–73.
9. Sunol A, Mascort J, Font C, et al. Long-term follow-up of surgical resection alone for primary intracranial rostrotentorial tumors in dogs: 29 cases (2002-2013). Open Vet J 2017;7(4):375–83.

10. Forward AK, Volk HA, Cherubini GB, et al. Clinical presentation, diagnostic findings and outcome of dogs undergoing surgical resection for intracranial meningioma: 101 dogs. BMC Vet Res 2022;18:88.
11. Ijiri A, Yoshiki K, Tsuboi S, et al. Surgical resection of twenty-three cases of brain meningioma. J Vet Med Sci 2014;76(3):331–8.
12. Edwards MR, Garcia Mora JK, Fowler KM, et al. Magnetic resonance and computed tomographic imaging characteristics and potential molecular mechanisms of feline meningioma associated calvarial hyperostosis. Vet Comp Oncol 2024;1–12. https://doi.org/10.1111/vco.12964.
13. Cameron S, Rishniw M, Miller AD, et al. Characteristics and survival of 121 cats undergoing excision of intracranial meningiomas (1994-2011). Vet Surg 2015;44: 772–6.
14. Pons-Sorolla M, Dominguez E, Czopowicz M, et al. Clinical and magnetic resonance imaging (MRI) features, tumour localisation, and survival of dogs with presumptive brain gliomas. Vet Sci 2022;9:257.
15. Bentley RT, Ober CP, Anderson KL, et al. Canine intracranial gliomas: relationship between magnetic resonance imaging criteria and tumor type and grade. Vet J 2013;198:463–71.
16. Diangelo L, Cohen-Gadol A, Heng HG, et al. Glioma mimics: magnetic resonance imaging characteristics of granulomas in dogs. Front Vet Sci 2019;28. https://doi.org/10.3389/fvets.2019.00286.
17. Jose-Lopez R, Gutierrez-Quintana R, de la Fuente C, et al. Clinical features, diagnosis, and survival analysis of dogs with glioma. J Vet Intern Med 2021;35: 1902–17.
18. Moirano SJ, Dewey CW, Wright KZ, et al. Survival times in dogs with presumptive intracranial gliomas treated with oral lomustine: A comparative retrospective study (2008-2017). Vet Comp Oncol 2018;16:459–66.
19. Bentley RT, Yanke AB, Miller MA, et al. Cerebrospinal fluid drop metastases of canine glioma: magnetic resonance imaging classification. Front Vet Sci 2021; 8. https://doi.org/10.3389/fvets.2021.650320.
20. Rissi DR, Miller AD. Feline glioma: a retrospective study and review of the literature. J Feline Med Surg 2017;19(12):1307–14.
21. MacLellan JD, Arnold SA, Dave AC, et al. Association of magnetic resonance imaging-based preoperative tumor volume with postsurgical survival time in dogs with primary intracranial glioma. J Am Vet Med Assoc 2018;252:98–102.
22. Mandara MT, Motta L, Calo P. Distribution of feline lymphoma in the central and peripheral nervous systems. Vet J 2016;216(6):109–16.
23. Durand A, Keenihan E, Schweizer, et al. Clinical and magnetic resonance imaging features of lymphoma involving the nervous system in cats. J Vet Intern Med 2022;36:679–93.
24. Siso S, Marco-Salazar P, Moore PF, et al. Canine nervous system lymphoma subtypes display characteristic neuroanatomical patterns. Vet Path 2017;54(1): 53–60.
25. LaRue MK, Taylor AR, Back AR, et al. Central nervous system lymphoma in 18 dogs (2001-2015). J Small Anim Pract 2018;59:547–52.
26. Lampe R, Levitin HA, Hecht S, et al. MRI of CNS lymphoma with choroid plexus involvement in five dogs and one cat. J Small Anim Pract 2021;62:690–9.
27. Mattei C, Oevermann A, Schweizer D, et al. MRI ischemic and hemorrhagic lesions in arterial and venous territories characterize central nervous system intravascular lymphoma in dogs. Vet Radiol Ultrasound 2023;64:294–305.

28. Mariani CL, Jennings MK, Olby NJ, et al. Histiocytic sarcoma with central nervous system involvement in dogs: 19 cases (2006-2012). J Vet Intern Med 2015;29: 607–13.
29. Toyoda I, Vernau W, Sturges BK, et al. Clinicopathological characteristics of histiocytic sarcoma affecting the central nervous system in dogs. J Vet Intern Med 2020;34:828–37.
30. Forward AK, Volk HA, De Decker S. Postoperative survival and early complications after intracranial surgery in dogs. Vet Surg 2018;47:549–54.
31. Morton BA, Selmic LE, Vitale S, et al. Indications, complications, and mortality rate following craniotomy or craniectomy in dogs and cats: 165 cases (1995-2016). J Am Vet Med Assoc 2022;260(9):1048–56.
32. Parker RL, Du J, Shinn RL, et al. Incidence, risk factors, and outcomes for early postoperative seizures in dogs with rostrotentorial brain tumors after intracranial surgery. J Vet Intern Med 2022;36:694–701.
33. Hu H, Barker A, Harcourt-Brown T, et al. Systematic review of brain tumor treatment in dogs. J Vet Intern Med 2015;29:1456–63.
34. Korner M, Roos M, Meier, et al. Radiation therapy for intracranial tumors in cats with neurological signs. J Feline Med Surg 2019;21(8):765–71.
35. Treggiari E, Maddox TW, Goncalves R, et al. Retrospective comparison of three-dimensional conformal radiation therapy vs. prednisolone alone in 30 cases of canine infratentorial brain tumors. Vet Radiol Ultrasound 2017;58(1):106–16.
36. Hansen KS, Li CF, Theon AP, et al. Stereotactic radiotherapy outcomes for intraventricular brain tumours in 11 dogs. Vet Comp Oncol 2023;21:665–72.
37. Zwingenberger AL, Pollard RE, Taylor SL, et al. Perfusion and volume response of canine brain tumors to stereotactic radiosurgery and radiotherapy. J Vet Intern Med 2016;30:827–35.
38. Bentley RT, Thomovsky SA, Miller MA, et al. Canine (pet dog) tumor microsurgery and intratumoral concentration and safety of metronomic chlorambucil for spontaneous glioma: a phase 1 clinical trial. World Neurosurg 2018;116:e534–42.
39. Crespo EH, Marine AF, Pumarola i Battle M, et al. Survival time after surgical debulking and temozolomide adjuvant chemotherapy in canine intracranial gliomas. Vet Sci 2022;9(8):427.
40. Duncan KL, Kuntz CA, Simcock JO. Transorbital craniectomy for treatment of frontal lobe and olfactory bulb neoplasms in two dogs. J Am Vet Med Assoc 2021;258(11):1236–42.
41. Doran CE, Frank CB, McGrath S, et al. Use of handheld Raman spectroscopy for intraoperative differentiation of normal brain tissue from intracranial neoplasms in dogs. Front Vet Sci 2022;26. https://doi.org/10.3389/fvets.2021.819200.
42. Carrera I, Richter H, Beckmann K, et al. Evaluation of intracranial neoplasia and noninfectious meningoencephalitis in dogs by use of short echo time, single voxel proton magnetic resonance spectroscopy at 3.0 Tesla. Am J Vet Res 2016;77(5):452–62.
43. Stadler KL, Ober CP, Feeney DA, et al. Multivoxel proton magnetic resonance spectroscopy of inflammatory and neoplastic lesions of the canine brain at 3.0 T. Am J Vet Res 2014;75:982–9.
44. Shinn RL, Kani Y, Hsu FC, et al. Risk factors for adverse events occurring after recovery from stereotactic brain biopsy in dogs with primary intracranial neoplasia. J Vet Intern Med 2020;34:2021–8.
45. Hanael E, Baruch S, Chai O, et al. Quantitative analysis of magnetic resonance images for characterization of blood-brain barrier dysfunction in dogs with brain tumors. J Vet Intern Med 2023;37:606–17.

46. Meyerhoff N, Volk HA, De Decker S, et al. Quantitative analysis of magnetic resonance images for characterization of blood-brain barrier dysfunction in dogs with brain tumors. J Vet Intern Med 2023;37:606–17.
47. Packer RA, Rossmeisl JH, Kent MS, et al. Consensus recommendations on standardized magnetic resonance imaging protocols for multicenter canine brain tumor clinical trials. Vet Radiol Ultrasound 2018;59:261–71.
48. Garcia PA, Kos B, Rossmeisl JH, et al. Predictive therapeutic planning for irreversible electroporation treatment of spontaneous malignant glioma. Med Phys 2017;44(9):4968–80.
49. Ammons DT, Guth A, Rozental AJ, et al. Reprogramming the canine glioma microenvironment with tumor vaccination plus oral losartan and propranolol induces objective responses. Cancer Res Commun 2022;2(12):1657–67.
50. Boudreau CE, Najem H, Ott M, et al. Intratumoral delivery of STING agonist results in clinical responses in canine glioblastoma. Clin Cancer Res 2021;27: 5528–35.
51. Chambers MR, Foote JB, Bentley RT, et al. Evaluation of immunologic parameters in canine glioma patients treated with an oncolytic herpes virus. J Transl Genet Genom 2021;5(4):423–42.
52. Olin MR, Ampudia-Mesias E, Pennell CA, et al. Treatment combining CD200 immune checkpoint inhibitor and tumor-lysate vaccination after surgery for pet dogs with high-grade glioma. Cancers 2019;11:137.
53. Sayour EJ, Grippin A, De Leon G, et al. Personalized tumor RNA loaded lipid-nanoparticles prime the systemic and intratumoral milieu for response to cancer immunotherapy. Nano Lett 2018;18:6195–206.
54. Cloquell A, Mateo I, Gambera S, et al. Systemic cellular viroimmunotherapy for canine high-grade gliomas. Journal for ImmunoTherapy of Cancer 2022;10: e005669.

Brain MRI Protocol and Systematic Approach to Interpretation of Brain Tumors on MRI

Samantha Loeber, DVM, DACVR, DACVR-EDI*

KEYWORDS

- Brain tumor • Intracranial neoplasia • Canine • Feline • Magnetic resonance imaging

KEY POINTS

- MRI remains the imaging modality of choice for the diagnosis of brain tumors in dogs and cats, with an overall high level of diagnostic accuracy.
- Consensus recommendations for brain tumor MRI protocols have been reported in an effort to enhance repeatability and consistency amongst institutions.
- A systematic approach to brain tumor evaluation on MRI with standard interpretation criteria may allow presumptive diagnosis, though limitations exist.

INTRODUCTION

MRI is the imaging modality of choice for evaluation of brain tumors in veterinary patients. Excellent high-contrast soft-tissue resolution of MRI affords it to be an invaluable tool in neuro-oncology that is integral for noninvasive morphologic characterization of brain tumors. Imaging features of brain tumors on MRI are used to make a presumptive antemortem diagnosis and formulate a prioritized list of differential diagnoses. Lesion identification and accurate differentiation of tumor type is important for patient prognosis and decisions in treatment planning.

Primary brain neoplasia represents approximately 1.5% to 4.5% of all cancers in dogs and approximately 2.2% of all cancers in cats.[1–4] Characteristics of intracranial neoplasms on MRI of the dog and cat have been described in numerous retrospective case series and case reports. This body of literature tends to show that MRI findings of brain tumors often are non-specific and variable with overlapping features, making accurate antemortem diagnosis challenging. High-field MRI has been shown to be 94.4% sensitive and 95.5% specific for overall detection of brain lesions in dogs

Department of Surgical Sciences, University of Wisconsin-Madison, 2015 Linden Drive, Madison, WI 53706, USA
* 2015 Linden Drive, Madison, WI 53706.
E-mail address: SLoeber@wisc.edu

Vet Clin Small Anim 55 (2025) 11–21
https://doi.org/10.1016/j.cvsm.2024.07.003
0195-5616/25/© 2024 Elsevier Inc. All rights reserved, including those for text and data mining, AI training, and similar technologies.

with very good inter-rater agreement, particularly in the detection of neoplastic brain disease.[5] In a study of 41 dogs with histopathologically confirmed intracranial neoplasia, MRI was approximately 90% sensitive for detecting brain lesions; however, was only 70% sensitive in determining tumor type in dogs with primary brain neoplasia.[6] Sensitivity of MRI has been reported as consistently much lower than specificity for multiple tumor types, with the highest sensitivity associated with glioma and pituitary tumor (84.4% and 83.3%, respectively), compared to meningioma with a sensitivity of 64.9% to 100% depending on the study.[7] Sensitivity of MRI to correctly identify meningiomas in cats is reported to be up to 96%.[8,9] Specificity of brain MRI in dogs has been reported as high across multiple tumor types including glioma (93.7%–99.3%) and meningioma (up to 94.9%).[7] In a study evaluating feline primary intracranial neoplasia, reviewers correctly identified 82% of all tumor types based on MRI appearance alone.[9] Despite the high specificity of MRI, specific neoplastic brain diseases are frequently misclassified and differentiation of neoplastic from non-neoplastic diseases can be challenging.[7,10] A collection of literature has shown that basic MRI signal characteristics have been unreliable in differentiating tumor type, tumor grade, and disease category.[8,11–13]

MRI interpretation is inherently subjective and prone to observer variation, even amongst experienced practitioners. Radiologists have been found to be reasonably consistent and accurate for selecting a category of diagnosis when interpreting canine brain MRI studies.[14] Interobserver agreement has been reported as good when identifying a brain lesion on MRI, but substantially more variable for interpreting features such as hemorrhage, edema, and pattern of contrast enhancement (fair to moderate agreement), dural tail sign and categorization of margins of enhancement (fair to substantial agreement), and axial localization, presence of mass effect, cavitation, signal intensity, and distribution of enhancement (moderate to substantial agreement).[14] High performance of MRI for diagnosing canine intracranial disease has been suggested to be due to recognition of multiple imaging characteristics rather than relying on any 1 feature alone.[5] Limitations of MRI, ambiguous imaging features of brain tumors and other lesions, and aggressive nature of some intracranial neoplasms such as gliomas, warrant improvements in the MRI diagnosis of brain tumors including optimization of image acquisition protocols and methodical approach to brain tumor evaluation on MRI.

DISCUSSION
Brain MRI Protocol and Optimization for Brain Tumors

MRI of dogs and cats with brain tumors should be performed via a standardized imaging protocol that is uniform across major MRI system manufacturers and applicable to different magnetic field strength scanners for accurate and reproducible brain imaging. An optimized MRI protocol should address the clinical question, be complete, reproducible, have high image quality, and be as fast as possible. Magnetic resonance (MR) technologists must be trained to recognize the need to acquire additional sequences and consult an on-site radiologist or remote access real-time radiologist prior to study completion. Additional MRI sequence selection to ensure a complete, comprehensive study must be balanced with scan length and anesthesia time. Optimized brain MRI protocols are of particular importance, given that spontaneous canine brain tumors are increasingly recognized as a translational model for the study of brain tumors in human patients.[15]

A variety of MRI sequences are commonly used in brain protocols and vary with institution, clinician preference, and equipment manufacturer. Consensus recommendations on standardized canine brain tumor MRI protocols including sequence selection and image acquisition parameters have been proposed at 1.5T and 3T field strengths.[15] A rapid brain MRI protocol evaluated in 104 dogs and 14 cats resulted in comparable differential diagnoses for the abbreviated protocol compared to a standard brain protocol.[16] The proposed shortened protocol had an average scan duration of 33 minutes compared to the 50 minutes scan duration of the standard brain protocol. A summary of the proposed minimum recommended sequence protocols and rapid brain MRI protocol is listed in **Table 1**. Additional sequences should be performed based on clinical indication, tailored to suit the individual patient.

Proposed consensus recommendations for specific image acquisition parameters for canine brain MRI including field of view (FOV), slice thickness, and matrix size have been described.[15] A field of view ≤150 mm is recommended in all 3 planes for both 2-dimensional (2D) and 3-dimensional (3D) images. Images should be acquired perpendicular to the hard palate from rostral to the cribriform plate to mid-first cervical vertebra (C1).[17] Three-D T1-weighted (T1w) images should have isotropic voxels ≤ 1 mm, with no gap and no overlap. Slice thickness should be ≤3 mm for 2D brain imaging with 2 mm considered ideal to allow for better tumor delineation and to reduce volume averaging. However, thicker slices such as 4 mm (maximum 5 mm) may be necessary for adequate signal on 1.5T scanners.[18] Matrix size should be ≥256 (256 × 256) for 2D images. Higher MRI field strength results in improved spatial resolution, signal to noise ratio (SNR), and contrast to noise ratio relative to scan time; however, it should be noted that chemical shift and magnetic susceptibility artifacts can be more prevalent and problematic in higher fields such as 3T. Feline patients undergo brain MRI less frequently than dogs. Brain MRI protocol recommendations have not been specifically outlined for cats. The small size of feline patients necessitates smaller FOV and thinner slices resulting in lower SNR. Adjustments must be made to ensure adequate SNR and optimized image quality.

Approach to MRI Sequence Selection and Justification

Information about tumor structure, margination, vascularization, fluid content, peritumoral edema, and inflammation is assessed on routine MRI sequences.[19] T1w images are useful for anatomic definition. T1w gradient echo (GRE) has been reported to have superior gray/white matter distinction over T1w turbo spin echo (TSE) sequences.[20] A benefit of 3D T1w images proposed in the consensus recommendation is that they can be reconstructed in each plane without the need for additional MR acquisitions. Additionally, 3D isotropic images (eg, 1 mm × 1 mm × 1 mm) allow for detection of smaller lesions and tumor volume estimation. Post-contrast 2-dimensional (2D) T1w images may have increased contrast medium conspicuity compared to 3D T1w images; however, 3D T1w images perform similarly and may depict non-enhancing tumors better.[21,22] The selection of T1w 2D or 3D images may be an institutional or individual preference and based on the patient's clinical status with scan time in mind.

T2-weighted (T2w) sagittal images should be acquired early in the scan to allow for rapid assessment of anatomic structures and facilitate identification of transtentorial and foramen magnum herniation secondary to mass effect (**Fig. 1A**). T2w images are useful for lesion identification, clinical diagnosis, and monitoring of non-contrast-enhancing tumors.[17] T2w fluid-attenuated inversion recovery (FLAIR) suppresses signal from fluid including cerebrospinal fluid (CSF) and therefore increases lesion conspicuity, allows for lesion assessment adjacent to CSF filled structures, and allows for better visualization of vasogenic edema.[17] T2* gradient echo (GRE) is useful to assess for the presence of blood degradation products in hemorrhagic lesions due to ferric/ferrous ions in hemoglobin metabolites causing local field distortion

Table 1
Summary of consensus recommendations of minimum MRI protocol for canine brain tumors and proposed rapid brain MRI protocol

Protocol Name	Sequence Name						
Consensus Recommendations for Canine Brain Tumors[15]	T2w Sag (TSE/FSE)	3D T1w (pre-C)	T2*w GRE Trans	T2w FLAIR Trans (TSE/FSE)	2D DWI	T2w Trans (TSE/FSE)	3D T1w + C
Proposed Rapid Brain MRI Protocol[16]	T2w Sag TSE	T2w FLAIR Trans TSE	T2*w GRE Trans	T1w Trans SE	DWI/ADC	T1w Trans SE + C	

Abbreviations: +C, postcontrast medium administration; 2D, 2 dimensional; 3D, 3 dimensional; ADC, apparent diffused coefficient; DWI, diffusion weighted imaging; FLAIR = fluid-attenuated inversion recovery; FSE, fast spin echo; GRE, gradient echo; pre-C, pre-contrast; Sag, sagittal; SE, spin echo; T1w, T1-weighting; T2*w, T2*-weighting; T2w, T2-weighting; trans, transverse; TSE, turbo spin echo.

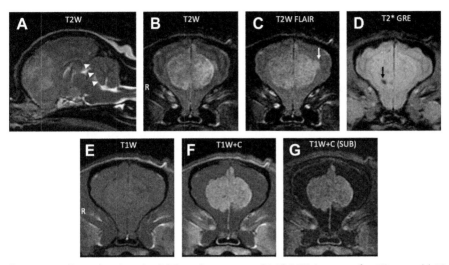

Fig. 1. Two-dimensional sagittal (*A*) and transverse (*B–G*) MRI images of a 12-year-old FS Shih Tzu with a bilateral falcine meningioma (transitional type). The T2w sagittal image is useful for identifying the presence of a mass effect resulting in transtentorial herniation (*A, white arrowheads*). A small amount of perilesional edema is best delineated on T2w fluid-attenuated inversion recovery (FLAIR) image (*C, white arrow*). Intralesional signal void/susceptibility artifact is identified on T2* GRE (*D, black arrow*). Note the strong, homogeneous contrast enhancement of the mass and utility of subtraction image for easy identification and delineation of contrast enhancement (*E-G*).

that appears as a signal void also known as susceptibility artifact.[23] (**Fig. 1**B–D) Diffusion-sensitive MRI techniques are routinely acquired as part of standard brain MRI protocols and are based on microscopic movement of water. Diffusion data are reported as apparent diffusion coefficient (ADC), a measure of the general magnitude of water motion. Lower ADC corresponds to decreased movement of water and restricted diffusion.[24,25] (**Fig. 2**) Restricted diffusion can occur in areas of tumor due to

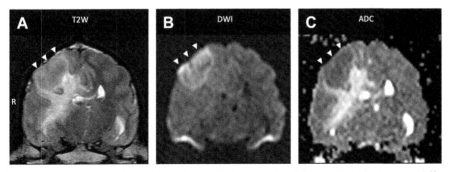

Fig. 2. Transverse T2-weighted (*A; T2w*), diffusion weighted (*B; DWI*), and apparent diffusion coefficient (*C; ADC*) MRI images of a 10-year-old FS Pit Bull mix with an intracranial extra-axial histiocytic sarcoma of the right parietal lobe (*arrowheads*). The mass is heterogeneously hyperintense on T2w and diffusion weighted images, and hypointense on apparent diffusion coefficient corresponding to decreased movement of water and restricted diffusion.

tightly packed tumor cells and increased cellular density and may result in lower ADC values.[10,23,24] In human brain tumors, ADC has shown to be a surrogate for cellularity in certain circumstances, with ADC inversely correlated with tumor cell density.[24–28] In contrast, necrosis, cellular lysis, and edema will increase ADC values due to expansion of extracellular fluid compartment volume that facilitates movement of water.

Intravenous (IV) contrast administration is recommended in all brain MRI studies for improved lesion detection, delineation, and characterization.[14,15,18,19] Parameter-matched pre-contrast and post-contrast sequences should be performed to allow for subtraction images. Subtraction images are recommended, when possible,[15] and can be performed automatically on most commercial image analysis platforms. By subtracting voxel intensities obtained on pre-contrast T1w images from post-contrast T1w images, contrast accumulation can be more easily identified and quantified.[18] (**Fig. 1**E–G) Contrast medium agent, dosing, and timing of administration should be standardized when possible. A dose of 0.1 mmol/kg IV gadolinium contrast medium that shortens T1 relaxation time is recommended. Optimal duration between contrast medium injection and image acquisition has not been defined in dogs and cats; however, a delay of 3 to 5 minutes has been proposed, and a delay of at least 5 minutes appears beneficial.[15] Quality control of post-contrast MR images with confirmation of readily apparent contrast enhancement of the normal choroid plexus, meningeal blood vessels, and nasal mucosa should be performed on every study. Regional lymph nodes and salivary glands included in the FOV should also be readily identified as contrast enhancing structures. If additional T1w post-contrast sequences such as fast spin echo or TSE with chemical fat saturation for improved sensitivity of contrast enhancement are desired, it is recommended to perform these after the T1w 3D image acquisition, if 3D images are being performed.[15,18]

MRI Interpretation of Brain Tumors

A systematic approach to brain tumor evaluation on MRI with standard interpretation criteria of imaging characteristics to allow for presumptive diagnosis has been described (**Table 2**).[5,11,29] Brain tumors are generally characterized as intra-axial or extra-axial dependent upon their origin of inside or outside of brain parenchyma and relationship with the subarachnoid space. Intraventricular tumors are commonly defined as extra-axial, though have been categorized as intra-axial or placed in their own intraventricular category.[12,30,31] It is important to differentiate extra-axial from intra-axial lesion origin to facilitate accurate prioritization of differential diagnoses. Extra-axial lesion location is suggested by broad-based meningeal contact, a mass that forms an obtuse angle with the surface of the adjacent brain, may widen the subarachnoid space, and display a "dural tail sign" on post-contrast images. A dural tail sign, defined as linear meningeal thickening and enhancement adjacent to and in continuity with a peripherally located cranial mass,[32] has been reported as a common MRI feature of extra-axial neoplasia, reported to be observed in 9% of all canine intracranial neoplasms, and 36% of meningiomas in dogs.[5] Dural tail sign had a predictive value of 94% for neoplasia in dogs and cats in a study[11] and is a common finding in meningioma; however, it is not specific to meningioma and has been described with other neoplasms and inflammatory conditions.[11,32–35] Intra-axial lesion location occurs inside the brain parenchyma and is suggested by formation of an acute angle with the surface of the adjacent brain and absence of adjacent meningeal enhancement.[36,37] Normal brain is typically evident between the lesion and the neurocranium. A "claw sign," defined as occurring when an expansile lesion within an organ creates thinning of the surrounding parenchyma generating a "claw-like" appearance, has been used to aid in the differentiation of intra-axial and extra-axial lesions, particularly

Table 2
Criteria for systematic approach to evaluating brain tumors on MRI

Criteria	Description
Tumor Origin	Intra-axial
	Extra-axial
	Intraventricular
Tumor Shape	Round
	Ovoid
	Lobulated
	Amorphous
Margination	Smooth
	Irregular
	Well-defined
	Poorly defined
Signal intensity (*to normal gray matter*) and Uniformity	*T2w, T1w, FLAIR*
	Hyperintense
	Hypointense
	Isointense
	Homogeneous
	Heterogeneous
T2* GRE Signal Voids	Yes or No
Degree and pattern of Contrast enhancement	None
	Mild
	Moderate
	Strong
	Homogeneous
	Heterogeneous
	Ring enhancing
	Other
Presence of mass effect	Yes or No
Peritumoral edema presence and degree	None
	Peritumoral
	Extensive

in the differentiation of meningiomas and peripherally occurring contrast-enhancing gliomas.[37] (**Fig. 3**).

Tumor shape, margination, T2w, T1w, and FLAIR signal intensity, and uniformity (homogeneous vs heterogeneous) should be noted. The tumor should be evaluated for the presence of T2* GRE signal voids, the degree and pattern of contrast enhancement, the presence of a mass effect, and for peritumoral edema. Seven MRI characteristics have been reported to be predictive of brain neoplasia in dogs and cats including a single lesion, regular shape (spheroidal, ovoidal), presence of mass effect, dural contact, dural tail sign, lesions affecting adjacent bone, and contrast enhancement.[11] The presence of contrast enhancement on MRI has a predictive value for neoplasia of 74% in dogs and cats.[11] Strong contrast enhancement is a common feature of some brain tumors including meningioma, lymphoma, choroid plexus tumors, and high-grade gliomas.[1,6,12,13,38,39] In a study assessing MRI characteristics to differentiate neoplastic, inflammatory, and vascular brain lesions in 75 dogs,[5] strong contrast enhancement was the single MRI characteristic that occurred at a slightly higher frequency in neoplasia than other diseases in the study group. However, the presence of lesion contrast enhancement was seen equally among neoplastic, inflammatory, and vascular categories. Therefore, contrast enhancement alone is not an

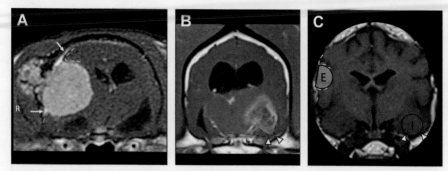

Fig. 3. Transverse T1w post-contrast MRI images (*A, B*) and schematic MRI diagram (*C*) demonstrating features of intra-axial and extra-axial mass locations. (*A*) Extra-axial mass (transitional meningioma in 11-year-old MN DSH) defined by broad-based meningeal contact, a mass that forms an obtuse angle with the surface of the brain (yellow dashed *lines*), and a dural tail sign (*white arrows*). Skull infiltration and extra-cranial extension are noted in this case. (*B*) Intra-axial mass (grade III oligodendroglioma in 4.5-year-old MN Boxer) demonstrating a "claw sign" defined as thinning of the surrounding brain parenchyma with a "claw-like" appearance that creates an acute angle with a sharp point (red dashed *lines,* white *arrowheads*). (*C*) Schematic demonstrating characteristics of extra-axial (E, yellow) and intra-axial (I, red) mass locations. A "claw sign" is delineated by the red dashed lines and white arrowheads.

indicator of neoplasia. A mass effect with a shift of brain parenchyma or compression of the ventricular system is a common feature of brain tumors;[30,40] however, is not specific to neoplasia and has been reported to occur in up to 65% of cases with cerebrovascular disease in dogs, most commonly with hemorrhagic infarcts.[5]

SUMMARY

MRI is an invaluable diagnostic tool for the evaluation of brain tumors in dogs and cats. Standard MRI sequences allow feature analysis to discriminate lesion types and formulate prioritized lists of differential diagnoses; however, overlapping imaging features make presumptive diagnosis based on diagnostic imaging alone challenging. The pathologic similarities between canine and human primary brain tumors have been well established, and there is interest in using naturally occurring brain tumors in dogs as a translational model for advancing treatment options in both animals and human patients.

CLINICS CARE POINTS

- Standardization of brain MRI protocol is useful for obtaining efficient, high-quality, repeatable diagnostic imaging studies in dogs and cats. Consensus recommendations should be referenced when designing and revising MRI protocols.

- A structured, systematic approach to MRI evaluation of brain tumors in dogs and cats is important to allow for an accurate presumptive diagnosis and prioritized differential diagnoses.

DISCLOSURE

The author has no commercial or financial conflicts of interest to disclose.

REFERENCES

1. Snyder JM, Shofer FS, Van Winkle TJ, et al. Canine intracranial primary neoplasia: 173 cases (1986-2003). J Vet Intern Med 2006;20(3):669–75.
2. Song RB, Vite CH, Bradley CW, et al. Postmortem evaluation of 435 cases of intracranial neoplasia in dogs and relationship of neoplasm with breed, age, and body weight. J Vet Intern Med 2013;27(5):1143–52.
3. Miller AD, Miller CR, Rossmeisl JH. Canine Primary Intracranial Cancer: A Clinicopathologic and Comparative Review of Glioma, Meningioma, and Choroid Plexus Tumors. Front Oncol 2019 8;9:1151.
4. Zaki FA, Hurvitz AI. Spontaneous neoplasms of the central nervous system of the cat. J Small Anim Pract 1976;17(12):773–82.
5. Young BD, Fosgate GT, Holmes SP, et al. Evaluation of standard magnetic resonance characteristics used to differentiate neoplastic, inflammatory, and vascular brain lesions in dogs. Vet Radiol Ultrasound 2014;55(4):399–406.
6. Rodenas S, Pumarola M, Gaitero L, et al. Magnetic resonance imaging findings in 40 dogs with histologically confirmed intracranial tumours. Vet J 2011;187(1): 85–91.
7. Wolff CA, Holmes SP, Young BD, et al. Magnetic resonance imaging for the differentiation of neoplastic, inflammatory, and cerebrovascular brain disease in dogs. J Vet Intern Med 2012;26(3):589–97.
8. Troxel MT, Vite CH, Van Winkle TJ, et al. Feline intracranial neoplasia: retrospective review of 160 cases (1985-2001). J Vet Intern Med 2003;17(6):850–9.
9. Troxel MT, Vite CH, Massicotte C, et al. Magnetic resonance imaging features of feline intracranial neoplasia: retrospective analysis of 46 cats. J Vet Intern Med 2004;18(2):176–89.
10. Cervera V, Mai W, Vite CH, et al. Comparative magnetic resonance imaging findings between gliomas and presumed cerebrovascular accidents in dogs. Vet Radiol Ultrasound 2011;52(1):33–40.
11. Cherubini GB, Mantis P, Martinez TA, et al. Utility of magnetic resonance imaging for distinguishing neoplastic from non-neoplastic brain lesions in dogs and cats. Vet Radiol Ultrasound 2005;46(5):384–7.
12. Kraft SL, Gavin PR, Dehaan C, et al. Retrospective review of 50 canine intracranial tumors evaluated by magnetic resonance imaging. J Vet Intern Med 1997;11: 218–25.
13. Young BD, Levine JM, Porter BF, et al. Magnetic resonance imaging features of intracranial astrocytomas and oligodendrogliomas in dogs. Vet Radiol Ultrasound 2011;52(2):132–41.
14. Leclerc MK, d'Anjou MA, Blond L, et al. Interobserver agreement and diagnostic accuracy of brain magnetic resonance imaging in dogs. J Am Vet Med Assoc 2013;242(12):1688–95.
15. Packer RA, Rossmeisl JH, Kent MS, et al. Consensus recommendations on standardized magnetic resonance imaging protocols for multicenter canine brain tumor clinical trials. Vet Radiol Ultrasound 2018;59(3):261–71.
16. Johnson KA, Sutherland-Smith J, Oura TJ, et al. Rapid brain MRI protocols result in comparable differential diagnoses versus a full brain protocol in most canine and feline cases. Vet Radiol Ultrasound 2023;64(1):86–94.
17. Robertson I. Optimal magnetic resonance imaging of the brain. Vet Radiol Ultrasound 2011;52(1 Suppl 1):S15–22.
18. Ellingson BM, Bendszus M, Boxerman J, et al, Jumpstarting Brain Tumor Drug Development Coalition Imaging Standardization Steering Committee. Consensus

recommendations for a standardized Brain Tumor Imaging Protocol in clinical trials. Neuro Oncol 2015;17(9):1188–98.

19. Johnson PJ, Rivard BC, Wood JH, et al. Relationship between histological tumor margins and magnetic resonance imaging signal intensities in brain neoplasia of dogs. J Vet Intern Med 2022;36(3):1039–48.

20. Komada T, Naganawa S, Ogawa H, et al. Contrast-enhanced MR imaging of metastatic brain tumor at 3 Tesla: utility of T(1)-weighted SPACE compared with 2D spin echo and 3D gradient echo sequence. Magn Reson Med Sci 2008;7:13–21.

21. Dodo T, Okada T, Yamamoto A, et al. T1-weighted MR imaging of glioma at 3T: A comparative study of 3D MPRAGE vs. conventional 2D spin-echo imaging. Clin Imaging 2016;40:12571261.

22. Zhu W, Qi J, Wang C. Comparative study of 3D-SPGR vs 2D-SE T1WI after enhancement in the brain. J Huazhong Univ Sci Technol - Med Sci 2003;23: 180–3.

23. Rossmeisl JH Jr, Garcia PA, Daniel GB, et al. Invited review–neuroimaging response assessment criteria for brain tumors in veterinary patients. Vet Radiol Ultrasound 2014;55(2):115–32.

24. Chenevert TL, Sundgren PC, Ross BD. Diffusion imaging: insight to cell status and cytoarchitecture. Neuroimaging Clin N Am 2006;16:619–32.

25. Ellingson BM, Malkin MG, Rand SD, et al. Validation of functional diffusion maps (fDMs) as a biomarker for human glioma cellularity. J Magn Reson Imag 2010; 31(3):538–48.

26. Sugahara T, Korogi Y, Kochi M, et al. Usefulness of diffusion-weighted MRI with echo-planar technique in the evaluation of cellularity in gliomas. J Magn Reson Imag 1999;9(1):53–60.

27. Chenevert TL, Stegman LD, Taylor JM, et al. Diffusion magnetic resonance imaging: an early surrogate marker of therapeutic efficacy in brain tumors. J Natl Cancer Inst 2000;92(24):2029–36.

28. Guo AC, Cummings TJ, Dash RC, et al. Lymphomas and high-grade astrocytomas: comparison of water diffusibility and histologic characteristics. Radiology 2002;224(1):177–83.

29. Jose-Lopez R, Gutierrez-Quintana R, de la Fuente C, et al. Clinical features, diagnosis, and survival analysis of dogs with glioma. J Vet Intern Med 2021;35(4): 1902–17.

30. Thomas WB, Wheeler SJ, Kramer R, et al. Magnetic resonance imaging features of primary brain tumors in dogs. Vet Radiol Ultrasound 1996;37:20–7.

31. Vural SA, Besalti O, Ilhan F, et al. Ventricular ependymoma in a German Shepherd dog. Vet J 2006;172(1):185–7.

32. Graham JP, Newell SM, Voges AK, et al. The dural tail sign in the diagnosis of meningiomas. Vet Radiol Ultrasound 1998;39(4):297–302.

33. Sturges BK, Dickinson PJ, Bollen AW, et al. Magnetic resonance imaging and histological classification of intracranial meningiomas in 112 dogs. J Vet Intern Med 2008;22(3):586–95.

34. Guermazi A, Lafitte F, Miaux Y, et al. The dural tail sign—beyond meningioma. Clin Radiol 2005;60:171–88.

35. Hathcock JT. Low field magnetic resonance imaging characteristics of cranial vault meningiomas in 13 dogs. Vet Radiol Ultrasound 1996;37:257–63.

36. Bentley RT. Magnetic resonance imaging diagnosis of brain tumors in dogs. Vet J 2015;205(2):204–16.

37. Glamann S, Jeffery ND, Levine JM, et al. The "Claw Sign" may aid in axial localization in cases of peripherally located canine glioma on MRI. Vet Radiol Ultrasound 2023;64(4):706–12.
38. Palus V, Volk HA, Lamb CR, et al. MRI features of CNS lymphoma in dogs and cats. Vet Radiol Ultrasound 2012;53(1):44–9.
39. Westworth DR, Dickinson PJ, Vernau W, et al. Choroid plexus tumors in 56 dogs (1985-2007). J Vet Intern Med 2008;22(5):1157–65.
40. Hecht S, Adams WH. MRI of brain disease in veterinary patients part 2: Acquired brain disorders. Vet Clin North Am Small Anim Pract 2010;40(1):39–63.

MRI Characteristics of Primary Brain Tumors and Advanced Diagnostic Imaging Techniques

Samantha Loeber, DVM, DACVR, DACVR-EDI*

KEYWORDS

- Intracranial neoplasia • Canine • Feline • Magnetic resonance imaging • Advanced

KEY POINTS

- There is an extensive body of literature describing magnetic resonance imaging characteristics of brain tumors in dogs and cats; however, a large degree of overlap between MRI features and different tumor types exists that can lead to misdiagnosis.
- Advanced diagnostic imaging techniques for brain tumor diagnosis, differentiation, and grading in dogs and cats are being explored and developed.
- The combination of conventional MRI and complementery advanced imaging techniques will likely provide optimized information for accurate patient diagnosis, prognostication, and targeted treatment development in veterinary medicine.

INTRODUCTION

Primary brain neoplasia represents approximately 1.5% to 4.5% of all cancers in dogs and approximately 2.2% of all cancers in cats.[1–4] Meningiomas are among the most common brain neoplasia and account for approximately 45% to 50% of primary intracranial neoplasms in dogs[1–3,5,6] and between 58% and 71% in cats.[7] Gliomas are the second most common primary brain tumor with a reported 30% to 40% incidence of all primary brain tumors in dogs,[1–3] but occur less frequently in cats making up approximately 8% of feline primary intracranial neoplasms.[7] The remaining cohort of tumors consist of a variety of less commonly occurring neoplasms including choroid plexus tumors (CPTs) (approximately 7% prevalence[3]), histiocytic sarcoma (up to 2.9% prevalence in dogs[1,2]), and lymphoma (2%–6% prevalence in dogs with a higher rate of occurrence in cats).[1,7–10]

MRI does not replace histopathological examination as a definitive means of phenotypic characterization of brain tumors, and brain biopsy remains fundamental for brain

Department of Surgical Sciences, University of Wisconsin-Madison, 2015 Linden Drive, Madison, WI 53706, USA
* Corresponding author.
E-mail address: SLoeber@wisc.edu

Vet Clin Small Anim 55 (2025) 23–39
https://doi.org/10.1016/j.cvsm.2024.07.004   vetsmall.theclinics.com
0195-5616/25/© 2024 Elsevier Inc. All rights reserved, including those for text and data mining, AI training, and similar technologies.

tumor diagnosis. Due to risk of complications and costs associated with obtaining brain biopsy samples, the importance of neuroimaging in disease classification is recognized.[11,12] Inherent limitations of MRI, overlapping imaging features of brain tumors with other diseases, and aggressive nature of some intracranial neoplasms such as gliomas, warrant improvements in the MRI diagnosis of brain tumors including development of advanced imaging techniques to allow advancements in patient care.

DISCUSSION
MRI Characteristics of Primary Canine and Feline Brain Tumors

MRI features of frequently occurring intra-axial and extra-axial brain tumors in dogs and cats have been described and a recent illustrated scoping review provides a comprehensive summary of MRI appearance and diagnostic approach to brain tumors in dogs and cats.[13] This review herein will focus on the most frequently occurring primary brain tumors in dogs and cats including the most common extra-axial tumors: meningiomas, histiocytic sarcomas, and intraventricular tumors, and the most common intra-axial tumors: gliomas such as low-grade and high-grade oligodendroglioma, astrocytoma, and undefined glioma.

EXTRA-AXIAL TUMORS
Meningioma

Meningiomas typically are strongly contrast-enhancing, extra-axial lesions associated with a dural tail sign that may have well-defined borders with the brain and smooth or irregular margins.[5,14–17] (**Fig. 1**) They are commonly single tumors, but multiple tumors can be present, especially in cats, with multiple meningiomas reported in up to 17% of all feline meningioma cases.[5,7,10,18,19] Meningiomas generally occur in domestic

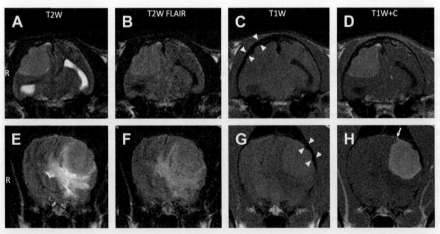

Fig. 1. Transverse MRI images of a 16-year-old male neutered domestic shorthair cat with a grade I transitional meningioma (top, *A–D*) and a 5-year-old female spayed goldendoodle with a grade II psammomatous meningioma (bottom, *E–H*). The feline meningioma is T2w and T2w fluid-attenuated inversion recovery (FLAIR) hyperintense, T1w hypointense, and strongly homogeneously contrast enhancing. There is a mass effect, obstructive hydrocephalus, and minimal to absent perilesional edema. The canine meningioma is T2w and T2w FLAIR slightly hyperintense, T1w mildly hyperintense, and strongly homogeneously contrast enhancing with a dural tail sign (*arrow*). There is a mass effect and marked perilesional edema. Calvarial hyperostosis is present in both cases (*arrowheads*).

shorthair cats and dolicocephalic dog breeds, especially German shepherd dogs, golden retrievers, and Labrador retrievers, with no consistent sex predisposition in either species.[1,5] Two broad categories of canine meningiomas are recognized by the World Health Organization (WHO) histologic classification scheme.[3,6,20] These categories include 1. benign, slow-growing neoplasms represented by 8 subtypes, most commonly: meningothelial, fibrous, transitional including psammomatous, and atypical, and 2. More anaplastic tumors with less benign behavior. Meningiomas are classified further into 3 histologic grades (WHO grade I–III), with benign, slow growing (WHO grade I) being more common than atypical meningioma (WHO grade II) and malignant or anaplastic meningioma (WHO grade III). Biological behavior of meningiomas in dogs and cats is generally considered benign, except for the anaplastic type.[6] The majority of feline meningiomas are WHO grade I, while in dogs atypical (grade II) meningiomas have a higher prevalence at >40% compared to benign meningioma which occurs 40% to 57% of the time.[6] Despite the relatively high sensitivity of MRI for the diagnosis of meningiomas, meningioma subtype or grade cannot be distinguished with conventional MRI sequences.[5] However, a study demonstrated the utility of apparent diffusion coefficient (ADC) values to differentiate atypical and malignant meningiomas from benign tumors, with atypical and malignant meningiomas displaying significantly lower ADC values compared to benign grade I meningiomas.[21]

Meningiomas are most commonly T2weigthed (w) and T2w fluid-attenuated inversion recovery (FLAIR) heterogeneously hyperintense (T2w hypointensity occurring in only 2% of meningiomas), T1w isointense or hypointense, and often display marked contrast enhancement.[5,6,10,17] Up to 20% of meningiomas can be T1w hyperintense pre-contrast, but the majority (70%) are T1w isointense.[3] They are usually well-defined and ovoid or spherical in shape, but can have a plaque-like conformation along the bony skull-base.[5,17] Meningiomas often cause a noticeable mass effect unless they are small in size and are frequently associated with peritumoral edema.[3,17] The majority of meningiomas are supratentorial in location, especially located in the fronto-olfactory region, but can also occur along the floor of the cranial cavity, the optic chiasm, suprasellar and parasellar regions, the cerebello-pontomedullary region and in cats, the third ventricle in the tela choroidea region.[1,5,6,10,14,16,17,22,23] Identification of cystic regions in meningeal masses may increase the suspicion of meningioma over other neoplasms, with cystic meningiomas most commonly occurring in the rostral cranial fossa.[5,24] Approximately 25% of canine meningiomas can have cystic or polycystic characteristics,[5,17,24] however, only 6% of feline meningiomas are reported to be cystic.[10] A dural tail sign is typically present in approximately 35% of meningiomas in dogs and in a study assessing MRI signs associated with intracranial neoplasia 82% of meningiomas in dogs and cats had a dural tail sign.[3,9] Approximately 50% to 70% of feline intracranial meningiomas are associated with a dural tail sign and calvarial hyperostosis, with calvarial hyperostosis reported in up to 73% of cats and 25% of dogs with meningioma.[10,16,18] Calvarial hyperostosis typically results in transdiploic bone thickening, sclerosis, and loss of diploic fat signal on MRI. Meningiomas can also cause lysis of bone adjacent to the tumor and have been reported to sporadically penetrate the cribriform plate causing confusion on MRI with olfactory neuroblastoma/esthesioneuroblastoma.[16,17,25] Intratumoral magnetic susceptibility artifact consistent with hemorrhage or mineralization has been reported in up to 40% of cats with meningiomas.[18]

Histiocytic Sarcoma

Intracranial histiocytic sarcoma (HS) is the most common solitary meningeal-based contrast-enhancing mass lesion after meningioma.[2,17,26] Histiocytic sarcoma is a histiocytic proliferative disorder with a localized, focal mass form and a disseminated/diffuse form[26,27] that can be poorly or well-defined, single or multifocal, intra-axial or extra-axial with extra-axial form being more common.[1,17,26,28,29] Meningiomas and HS share imaging features and typically show similar amounts of contrast enhancement and peritumoral edema.[30,31] Histiocytic sarcoma generally carries a worse prognosis than meningioma;[28,29] therefore, the ability to differentiate these tumors on MRI has clinical value.

Histiocytic sarcoma tends to be T2w hyperintense, T1w isointenseto hypointense, and moderately to strongly contrast enhancing, with a dural tail sign commonly observed.[1,3,17,22,26] Histiocytic sarcoma may display T2w isointensity or hypointensity more commonly than meningiomas.[31] In a study investigating the ability of MRI features to differentiate histiocytic sarcoma and meningioma in 51 dogs,[23] there was moderate interobserver agreement and good accuracy for differentiation of these tumors with good to excellent radiologist performance for the correct diagnosis using conventional MRI pulse sequences. Meningiomas more commonly had a broad-based appearance toward the neurocranium, cyst-like changes, osseous changes such as sclerosis/thickening of the adjacent neurocranium, and perilesional and pachymeningeal enhancement compared to HS. Histiocytic sarcoma tended to have more extensive edema and more often had combined perilesional and distant meningeal enhancement affecting both the pachymeninges and leptomeninges. These findings were similar to a study evaluating canine HS and meningiomas[30] that also found that all of the HS had leptomeningeal enhancement and mass invading into the sulci, providing more evidence that this is an important distinguishing feature between meningioma and HS (**Fig. 2**). Recent studies have suggested that transtentorial herniation and cranial cervical syringohydromyelia may be more prevalent with HS than meningioma indicating the more rapidly growing, aggressive nature of HS, though other studies have not reported this as a significant differentiation between HS and meningiomas.[28,30] Statistical differences in MRI diffusibility measurements for meningiomas and histiocytic sarcomas have been reported in a small sample of dogs.[30] In this study, intratumoral ADC values were significantly lower in HS than meningioma, potentially correlating with higher cellularity or grade of malignancy of HS compared to meningioma. The lack of blood vessel displacement on 3-dimensional (3D) time of flight magnetic resonance angiography in canine HS is another feature that may be useful in differentiating HS from meningioma in dogs.[31]

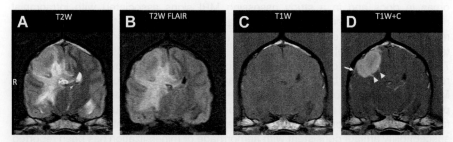

Fig. 2. Transverse MRI images of a 10-year-old female spayed pit bull mix with an intracranial extra-axial histiocytic sarcoma (*A–D*). The mass is heterogeneously T2w and FLAIR hyperintense, T1w slightly hypointense, and strongly, mildly heterogeneously contrast enhancing with a dural tail sign (*arrow*). The mass has tendrils of contrast enhancement that extend deeper into the parenchyma and within the sulci (*arrowheads*). There is a mass effect and marked perilesional edema.

Intraventricular Tumors

Intraventricular tumors may be located anywhere in the ventricular system including the lateral ventricles, interventricular foramen, third ventricle, mesencephalic aqueduct, fourth ventricle, or lateral apertures. The most common intraventricular tumors in dogs are CPTs such as papillomas and carcinomas, and less frequently ependymomas.[2,7,17,32] Third ventricular meningioma is the most common intraventricular tumor in cats followed by ependymoma, glioma, and CPT.[7,32] Mass replacing normal choroid plexus is more likely to be CPT than ependymoma. If normal choroid plexus can be identified separate from a ventricular mass, ependymoma should be considered.[17,22,33]

There is no accepted canine grading scheme for choroid plexus tumors; therefore, these tumors are commonly graded according to WHO human CPT criteria.[3] Choroid plexus papillomas are comparable to WHO grade I and are morphologically benign. Choroid plexus carcinomas are comparable to WHO grade III, are more histologically abnormal, and more likely to invade adjacent brain tissue or metastasize.[22] Ependymomas are often benign and do not tend to metastasize. They are divided into well-differentiated (WHO grade II) or anaplastic and aggressive (WHO grade III) categories.[22,32]

The majority of CPTs are located in the fourth ventricle (50%) followed by the third ventricle (22%–36%) and lateral ventricles (18%–29%),[11,22,34] while ependymomas most commonly occur in the rostral horn of the lateral ventricles.[14,17,33] Most CPTs have well-defined margins, cause obstructive ventriculomegaly, and approximately 50% will have periventricular edema.[3,17,33] Mild to moderate edema has been more frequently reported in choroid plexus carcinomas (70%) compared to choroid plexus papillomas (45%).[33] Some intraventricular tumors may be associated with incomplete suppression of cerebrospinal fluid (CSF) on T2w FLAIR images due to inflammation or increased protein content in the CSF.[32] CPTs are typically T2w hyperintense and can be T1w hyperintense, isointense, or hypointense, and are usually strongly contrast enhancing.[3,14,17,33] Choroid plexus carcinoma can display drop metastases to other ventricular and subarachnoid locations with a 33% incidence.[3,17] Identification of drop metastasis is a reliable means to differentiate a choroid plexus carcinoma from papilloma.[3] CPT in the fourth ventricle at the cerebellopontomedullary angle can be confused with meningiomas due to overlapping imaging features.[11,17]

Ependymomas are predominantly intraventricular masses derived from the lining of the epithelium of the ventricles, although they can invade the adjacent brain parenchyma with intra-axial and periventricular appearances.[14,17,22,35] A study evaluating the features of ependymomas in 5 cats described that all cats had obstructive hydrocephalus, transtentorial, and foramen magnum herniation.[32] CPTs and ependymomas share imaging features (**Fig. 3**), with ependymomas typically being moderately to markedly T2w and T2w FLAIR hyperintense, slightly T1w isointense, hypointense to slightly hyperintense with absent or minimal peritumoral edema.[14,22,36] Contrary to CPTs which are typically strongly contrast enhancing, ependymomas have more variable contrast enhancement from none to strong. Some CPTs and ependymomas have been reported to have cystic structures within them.[14,17,33]

INTRA-AXIAL TUMORS

Glioma

Gliomas are intra-axial tumors that vary greatly in appearance from poorly to well defined and may or may not display contrast enhancement.[3,37–39] A comprehensive grading system for canine gliomas exists[40] and 3 main glioma subtypes have been defined in dogs: oligodendroglioma (70% incidence), astrocytoma (20% incidence),

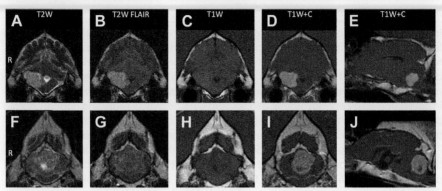

Fig. 3. Transverse (*A–D*) (*F–I*) and sagittal (*E, J*) MRI images of a 6.5-year-old male intact Labrador retriever with a choroid plexus papilloma of the lateral aperture of the fourth ventricle (top, A-E) and a 10-year-old male intact Alaskan malamute with an ependymoma of the caudal fossa (bottom, F-J). The choroid plexus papilloma was strongly T2w and T2w FLAIR hyperintense, T1w slightly hypointense, and strongly homogeneously contrast enhancing with mass effect and minimal perilesional edema. The ependymoma was heterogeneously T2w hyperintense, slightly T2w FLAIR hyperintense, T1w hypointense, strongly heterogeneously contrast enhancing with mass effect, moderate perilesional edema, and obstructive hydrocephalus. In both cases, meningioma was incorrectly prioritized as the top differential diagnosis, given the overlapping imaging features between lateral aperture CPTs and cerebellopontine meningiomas and between caudal fossa meningiomas and ependymomas. The ependymoma was adhered to the cerebellum and the overlying dura at surgery. Parenchymal invasion couldn't be determined on histopathology due to small sections from surgical biopsy.

and undefined glioma (10% incidence). Gliomas are further divided into low or high grade based on a histologic grading scheme. Oligodendroglial and high-grade tumors are the most prevalent in dogs.[38,40] Over 50% of all gliomas in dogs occur in brachycephalic breeds.[2,38,40] In a recent study characterizing canine gliomas,[38] 78% of the dogs with gliomas were brachycephalic breed with boxers and bulldogs (French > English) overrepresented. A male sex predilection in canine gliomas has been reported with an incidence rate ratio of 1.53 for all males/females.[40] Location of gliomas is mainly in the forebrain most commonly in the fronto-olfactory, temporal, and parietal regions[37–39] with no association between glioma location and tumor grade in a recent study.[38] The piriform lobe is an overrepresented location for both high-grade and low-grade oligodendrogliomas.[40]

Gliomas have a widely variable MRI appearance among different types and grades with overlapping imaging features that cause confusion with other diseases such as cerebrovascular accident, inflammatory disease, and meningioma.[3,8,17,22,39] Up to 12% of meningiomas are reportedly misclassified as an intra-axial lesion due to peripherally located contrast-enhancing gliomas mimicking meningiomas.[8] A "claw sign" has been determined to be supportive but not pathognomonic for intra-axial localization of canine gliomas with a sensitivity of 85.5% and specificity of 80%, and proved useful for differentiating peripherally located contrast-enhancing gliomas from meningiomas.[41] Gliomas and cerebrovascular accidents have overlapping features including mass effect, perilesional edema, and ring contrast enhancement that have led to misinterpretation, with as many as 12% of gliomas incorrectly classified as infarcts and as many as 47% of cerebrovascular accidents misdiagnosed as gliomas.[42,43] Gliomas are generally significantly larger than presumed cerebrovascular accidents, and more commonly associated with mass effect (100% in gliomas, 24% in cerebrovascular accident) and perilesional edema.[43] Gliomas can cause restricted diffusion similar to ischemia with infarcts; however, ADC hyperintensity is significantly more common in gliomas, consistent with T2 shine-through effect, and acute infarcts may have lower ADC than neoplasia.[43,44] When diffusion-weighted imaging (DWI) is provided, the rate of misdiagnosis between cerebrovascular accident and glioma is much lower.[43]

The majority of gliomas have non-specific signal intensity and are generally characterized by a T2w isointense to hyperintense (90% hyperintense), T1w iso-intense to hypointense (80% isointense), frequently heterogeneous mass with varying degree of contrast enhancement ranging from none to strong with uniform, nonuniform, and ring-enhancing patterns and associated peritumoral edema.[1,3,14,17,37,39] **(Fig. 4)** Astrocytomas have been reported to be much more T1w isointense or hyperintense than oligodendrogliomas which have been reported to be more T1w hypointense.[38,39]

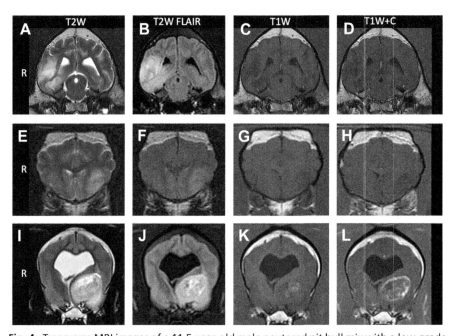

Fig. 4. Transverse MRI images of a 11.5-year-old male neutered pit bull mix with a low-grade oligodendroglioma (top, A–D), a 10-year-old male neutered French bulldog with a grade III oligodendroglioma (middle, E–H), and a 4.5-year-old male neutered Boxer with a grade III oligodendroglioma (bottom, I–L). Variable and overlapping imaging features are noted between these low-grade and high-grade tumors. The top tumor (A-D) is amorphous in shape, strongly T2w and T2w FLAIR hyperintense, T1w hypointense, and minimally to non-contrast enhancing. There is a mild mass effect with ventricular distortion. The middle tumor (E-H) is amorphous to lobular in shape, heterogeneously mildly T2w and T2w FLAIR hyperintense, T1w hypointense, and non-contrast enhancing. There is minimal mass effect with mild lateral ventricle compression. The bottom tumor (I-L) is rounded in shape, heterogeneously strongly T2w and T2w FLAIR hyperintense, T1w heterogeneously mixed T1w signal intensity with T1w hypointense, isointense, and hyperintense regions consistent with intralesional hemorrhage, and heterogeneously contrast enhancing with a peripheral contrast enhancing rim. There is mass effect with ventricular distortion and hydrocephalus. This tumor was displaying invasiveness on histology with necrosis and hemorrhage.

Gliomas often display a mass effect, reported in over 90% of astrocytomas and oligo-dendrogliomas.[37,39] Oligodendrogliomas are more commonly in contact with and distort ventricles than astrocytomas and have less peritumoral edema than astrocytomas.[17,37,38]

Contrast enhancement tends to be highly variable, with a ring-enhancing pattern often associated with gliomas.[40,43,45] Twenty-five percent of gliomas are non-contrast enhancing, and a lack of contrast enhancement is more likely with low-grade gliomas.[3] Low-grade gliomas have been reported to display lower degrees of contrast enhancement more commonly than high-grade gliomas; however, there can be poorly enhancing variants of high-grade glioma.[17,37,39] Of the gliomas that contrast enhance, 45% have partial or complete ring enhancement. Partial or complete ring contrast enhancement has been reported to occur in all grades of gliomas, with some studies reporting ring enhancement to be associated with high-grade gliomas and some studies finding no association with grade.[3,38,39,46–48] In some reports, nearly every glioblastoma (high-grade/grade 4 astrocytoma) was enhancing with moderate to marked enhancement.[37–39,48,49] Ring enhancement is not specific to gliomas and has been reported with several other neoplastic, vascular, and inflammatory brain diseases.[42,50]

Gliomas are composed of an inner core of solid tumor, surrounding penumbra of infiltrating tumor cells, and a region of edematous parenchyma on histopathology.[51] In a study assessing how MRI signal alterations relate to histologic tumor margins,[45] T2w, FLAIR, and T1w sequence signal intensity margins showed similarities to histologic margins for gliomas. These findings suggested that signal changes highlight the areas of infiltrating neoplastic penumbra, rather than solid tumor or perilesional edema alone, which is consistent with in people where fluid-rich T2w hyperintensity was found to include infiltrative neoplastic cells.[51–53] In that study, contrast enhancement did not correlate with histologic solid tumor margins and was consistently smaller in cross-sectional area than solid tumor margins. Therefore, margins of contrast enhancement alone should not be used for surgical or radiotherapy planning in gliomas.

Prediction of glioma type and grade using MRI features generally has low accuracy, limited sensitivity and specificity, high interobserver variability, and low agreement.[38] The T2w FLAIR mismatch signal (**Fig. 5**), described as lesions characterized by homogeneous T2w hyperintense signal that are T2w FLAIR hypointense (null signal) with a T2w FLAIR hyperintense peripheral rim, has been identified as an imaging marker for oligodendrogliomas in dogs.[54] The T2w FLAIR mismatch signal is uncommon in dogs with gliomas with a low sensitivity of 16%; however, when it is present, it has a reported 100% specificity for the detection of oligodendrogliomas and is significantly associated with non-enhancing low-grade oligodendrogliomas. Cystic regions tend to be more common in high-grade gliomas than low-grade gliomas.[17,39] Hemorrhage has been reported to occur in 30% to 40% of gliomas in all tumor types and grades but potentially more commonly in high grade.[17,37,39] In a recent study,[38] the only feature associated with a high-grade glioma was tumor spread to neighboring brain structures including drop metastasis. High-grade gliomas can infiltrate across the corpus callosum resulting in bihemispheric lesions that may have a symmetric, wing like appearance, termed "butterfly" glioma.[46] Butterfly glioma likely represents a pattern of spread rather than distinct type.[46,47] Canine butterfly glioma appears as a bihemispheric, intra-axial mass lesion that predominantly affects the corpus callosum and subcortical white matter of the frontoparietal regions and is associated with extensive perilesional edema and mass effect. Canine butterfly gliomas display heterogeneous T2w, T1w, and FLAIR signal intensities and variable contrast enhancement, with MRI characteristics similar to what has been described with glioblastoma multiforme.[46,48]

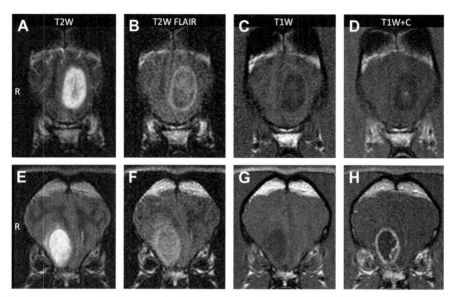

Fig. 5. Transverse MRI images of a 7.5-year-old male intact pit bull with an oligodendro-glioma (*top, A–D*) and a 7.5-year-old female spayed English bulldog with an oligodendro-glioma (*bottom, E–H*). Both tumors display T2w FLAIR mismatch signal characterized by homogeneous T2w hyperintensity and T2w FLAIR hypointensity with a T2w FLAIR hyperin-tense rim. Both tumors are strongly T2w hyperintense and T1w hypointense with a mass ef-fect. One has mild central contrast enhancement (*D*) and the other has strong peripheral rim contrast enhancement (*H*). Mild perilesional edema is present in the bottom case.

Gliomatosis cerebri is a rare, aggressive, tumor-like disease of glial cells character-ized by extensive, widespread neoplastic infiltration of brain parenchyma.[35,47,55–57] Signal abnormalities of the cerebral white and gray matter in at least 3 contiguous ce-rebral lobes with involvement of the thalamus and structures in the caudal fossa are suggestive of diffuse glioma with a gliomatosis cerebri growth pattern in dogs.[47,56] In a case series of 14 dogs with gliomatosis cerebri,[47] all lesions had severe changes with widespread growth pattern that presented as ill-defined intra-axial lesions within the left and right forebrain with involvement of the white and gray matter. Lesions were T2w and FLAIR hyperintense and T1w hypointense or isointense with minimal to mild contrast enhancement of the parenchyma and/or meninges. Gliomatosis cerebri may infiltrate without mass effect or have a solid tumor portion.[39,47,57–61] MRI can underes-timate gliomatosis cerebri lesions and some dogs with gliomatosis cerebri may have a normal MRI.[39]

Advanced diagnostic imaging techniques for brain tumors

Limitations of MRI in veterinary neuro-oncology have resulted in a body of literature dedicated to the investigation of functional and physiologic imaging that is considered complementary to conventional MRI. Sequences on MRI that provide functional and metabolic information about a tumor, improve the ability of MRI to discriminate be-tween neoplastic and non-neoplastic lesions, and predict tumor grade may be per-formed, but may not be developed enough for widespread clinical use.

Magnetic resonance spectroscopy is a noninvasive technique that evaluates brain biochemistry by quantifying the concentrations of specific metabolites from spectra of metabolite distributions to allow determination of tumor tissue.[62,63] Magnetic resonance spectroscopic metabolic signatures of a small number of canine brain tumors have been investigated and shown to parallel those of analogous human tumors.[64] Proton MR spectroscopy has been shown to be useful in the differentiation of canine intracranial neoplastic from non-neoplastic disease; however, no significant differences in metabolite spectra for canine meningiomas and gliomas have been detected.[62,63] Magnetic resonance spectroscopy may be beneficial as an adjunct to conventional MRI to diagnose and grade brain tumors in canine patients; however, more investigation is warranted.

Perfusion-weighted imaging involves serial acquisition of images in the same anatomic location during intravenous contrast administration to assess blood volume, perfusion, and permeability. Its applications have been investigated in people and dogs with brain tumors.[65–69] Two most commonly used techniques are dynamic susceptibility contrast and dynamic contrast-enhanced imaging. Dynamic susceptibility contrast generates maps of relative blood volume or flow in a target tissue and is referred to as relative cerebral (or tumor) blood volume and cerebral blood flow. Dynamic contrast-enhanced imaging is primarily used to assess capillary permeability.[65] In a study evaluating dynamic contrast enhanced MRI in a small number of dogs with different brain tumors,[69] there were statistical differences between distributions of enhancement pattern of each tumor, indicating a potential complementary technique to conventional MRI for noninvasive differentiation of brain tumor type in dogs.

Diffusion imaging techniques provide brain microstructural and functional information and aid in tumor characterization in human medicine.[70–72] Diffusion tensor imaging (DTI) provides additional information about the movement of water molecules in a 3D space and takes into account the direction of water diffusion in a particular voxel due to microstructure of underlying tissue.[70–72] Fractional anisotropy (FA) calculated from DTI is a quantitative index reflecting the magnitude of the oriented diffusion of water, and is considered to be associated with the architecture and integrity of white matter in the brain.[72] FA values relate to tumor consistency (softness or hardness) in human meningiomas, with a higher FA value indicating hard consistency tumor.[73] The FA value of feline meningiomas have been reported as significantly higher than canine meningiomas, correlating to typical firm consistency and benign behavior of most feline meningiomas compared to canine meningiomas which are often soft and fragile and tend to be more aggressive.[74,75] No significant difference was detected in intratumoral FA of histiocytic sarcomas and meningiomas in a small sample of dogs, indicating limited application of this technique for differentiation of these tumor types.[30] Diffusion imaging measurements may be affected by various factors such as density and composition of tumor cells, edema, and tumor necrosis; therefore, these metrics alone are not sufficient for the differentiation of tumors and future studies are needed to determine the sensitivity of these imaging characteristics.

PET is a functional imaging technique that has been used to evaluate intracranial neoplasia and is a well-established, routine clinical diagnostic imaging modality in human neuro-oncology.[76–82] It is a non-invasive, highly sensitive, advanced imaging technique for quantifying biologic function of tissue that uses radioactive tracers called radiopharmaceuticals to target specific biologic mechanisms in the body. It has poor resolution alone and thus is typically fused with computed tomography (CT) or MR images for anatomic localization. 2-deoxy-2-18F-fluorodeoxyglucose (18F-FDG) is the most common radiopharmaceutical used and reflects glucose metabolism throughout the body including brain tissue and/or tumors. FDG-PET has been developed and validated in human brain tumor patients[76–78] and has utility in grading gliomas in people when comparing lesion FDG avidity relative to gray and white matter.[79–82] High background activity in metabolically active normal brain tissue and limited FDG avidity of certain tumor types may be confounding in the use of FDG for brain tumors, so alternative tracers may be utilized. 18F-fluorothymidine is a marker for cell proliferation and has much lower uptake in normal brain tissue compared to FDG.[83,84] Amino acid PET such as C11-methionione (MET-PET) and 18F-fluoroethyltyrosine (FET-PET) has gained use in people due to high tumor to normal tissue contrast compared to FDG and its superior ability to FDG to define gross tumor volume and identify tumor recurrence in people with brain tumors.[83,85] These radiopharmaceuticals remain novel in veterinary medicine and have not yet been investigated in dogs and cats with brain tumors. FDG-PET of the brain has been evaluated in a variety of scenarios in dogs;[86–91] however, clinical use is not routine. FDG-PET MRI is currently being investigated in dogs with presumed intracranial neoplasia.[92] Case reports describing the use of PET in canine brain tumors are limited to a dog with intracranial histiocytic sarcoma imaged with FDG-PET[93] and a dog with a low-grade glioma imaged with FDG-PET and 3.4-dihydroxy-6-18F-fluoro-L-pheylala-nine (18F-FDOPA).[94] The canine intracranial histiocytic sarcoma revealed tumor hypermetabolism higher than gray matter on FDG-PET which correlated to malignancy on histopathology.[93] 18F-FDOPA PET revealed high lesion avidity in the canine glioma whereas tumor uptake was not detected on FDG-PET, indicating the potential utility of 18F-FDOPA in dogs with low FDG avidity brain tumors such as gliomas.[94]

The use of image texture analysis and deep learning techniques have been investigated in dogs with brain tumors.[95–98] Texture analysis via dedicated software quantifies tissue characteristics through feature extraction and evaluation of local image variations (eg, pixel signal intensity) on diagnostic imaging that may not be perceptible to the human eye. MRI texture-based radiomics has been shown to have a high accuracy for differentiating glioma from meningoencephalitis in dogs.[97] The features failed to differentiate canine glioma type and grade in a study;[97] however, the combination of MRI texture analysis and machine learning was able to differentiate canine glioma type and grade with 76% to 77% accuracy in a different study.[98] Deep learning via convolutional neural networks has been shown to have a high accuracy in discriminating between canine meningiomas and gliomas on MRI[96] and radiomic analysis of MR imaging features has shown the ability to discriminate grades of meningiomas in a small number of dogs.[95] Radiomics and machine learning techniques show promise in initial studies; however, limitations including availability and access to software, and variability and lack of standardization of interpretation techniques and methodology may limit widespread use and prohibit comparisons between institutions. Development of larger databases is needed to build predictive models for deep learning and texture analysis techniques for the analysis of brain tumors in dogs and cats on MRI.

SUMMARY

Conventional MRI allows imaging characteristic analysis to discriminate lesion types and formulate an accurate prioritized list of differential diagnoses; however, ambiguous imaging features make presumptive diagnosis based on MRI alone challenging. Advanced imaging techniques with quantitative MRI modalities will require further investigation and larger sample size to draw reasonable conclusions for clinical application in canine and feline brain tumor patients. The combination of conventional MRI with complementary advanced techniques will likely provide optimal information for patient diagnosis, prognostication, and treatment development in veterinary medicine.

CLINICS CARE POINTS

- MRI is relatively sensitive for differentiating brain tumor types in dogs and cats; however, challenges exist with overlapping MRI features between neoplastic and non-neoplastic lesions and between different neoplasms.
  - Large lesion size, the presence of mass effect, volume of perilesional edema, and DWI/ADC characteristics can be used to aid in the differentiation of gliomas from cerebrovascular accidents.
  - The "claw sign" may be used to determine intra-axial location in challenging cases of differentiating peripherally located contrast-enhancing gliomas from meningiomas.
  - Distant meningeal enhancement involving the leptomeninges in addition to the pachymeninges and more extensive edema can be used to differentiate histiocytic sarcomas from meningiomas.
- MRI features have a limited ability to differentiate glioma type and grade with high prevalence of overlapping imaging characteristics; however, criteria exist that increase the sensitivity/specificity/accuracy.
  - Oligodendroglioma should be prioritized with a more T1w hypointense intra-axial mass that has ventricular distortion.
  - Oligodendroglioma should be considered when T2w FLAIR mismatch is present.
  - Lack of contrast enhancement may indicate a low-grade glioma. Ring contrast enhancement can be seen in both grades but is more common in high-grade glioma.
- The identification of drop metastasis is most indicative of choroid plexus carcinoma when an intraventricular mass is present.
- Advanced MRI techniques are available complementary to conventional MRI but require further development for clinical application.

DISCLOSURE

The author has no commercial or financial conflicts of interest to disclose.

REFERENCES

1. Snyder JM, Shofer FS, Van Winkle TJ, et al. Canine intracranial primary neoplasia: 173 cases (1986-2003). J Vet Intern Med 2006 May-Jun;20(3):669–75.
2. Song RB, Vite CH, Bradley CW, et al. Postmortem evaluation of 435 cases of intracranial neoplasia in dogs and relationship of neoplasm with breed, age, and body weight. J Vet Intern Med 2013 Sep-Oct;27(5):1143–52.
3. Miller AD, Miller CR, Rossmeisl JH. Canine Primary Intracranial Cancer: A Clinicopathologic and Comparative Review of Glioma, Meningioma, and Choroid Plexus Tumors. Front Oncol 2019 Nov 8;9:1151.
4. Zaki FA, Hurvitz AI. Spontaneous neoplasms of the central nervous system of the cat. J Small Anim Pract 1976 Dec;17(12):773–82.
5. Sturges BK, Dickinson PJ, Bollen AW, et al. Magnetic resonance imaging and histological classification of intracranial meningiomas in 112 dogs. J Vet Intern Med 2008 May-Jun;22(3):586–95.
6. Motta L, Mandara MT, Skerritt GC. Canine and feline intracranial meningiomas: an updated review. Vet J 2012 May;192(2):153–65.
7. Troxel MT, Vite CH, Van Winkle TJ, et al. Feline intracranial neoplasia: retrospective review of 160 cases (1985-2001). J Vet Intern Med 2003 Nov-Dec;17(6): 850–9.

8. Young BD, Fosgate GT, Holmes SP, et al. Evaluation of standard magnetic resonance characteristics used to differentiate neoplastic, inflammatory, and vascular brain lesions in dogs. Vet Radiol Ultrasound 2014 Jul-Aug;55(4):399–406.
9. Cherubini GB, Mantis P, Martinez TA, et al. Utility of magnetic resonance imaging for distinguishing neoplastic from non-neoplastic brain lesions in dogs and cats. Vet Radiol Ultrasound 2005 Sep-Oct;46(5):384–7.
10. Troxel MT, Vite CH, Massicotte C, et al. Magnetic resonance imaging features of feline intracranial neoplasia: retrospective analysis of 46 cats. J Vet Intern Med 2004 Mar-Apr;18(2):176–89.
11. Heidner GL, Kornegay JN, Page RL, et al. Analysis of survival in a retrospective study of 86 dogs with brain tumors. J Vet Intern Med 1991;5:219–26.
12. Rossmeisl JH Jr, Garcia PA, Daniel GB, et al. Invited review–neuroimaging response assessment criteria for brain tumors in veterinary patients. Vet Radiol Ultrasound 2014 Mar-Apr;55(2):115–32.
13. May JL, Garcia-Mora J, Edwards M, et al. An Illustrated Scoping Review of the Magnetic Resonance Imaging Characteristics of Canine and Feline Brain Tumors. Animals 2024;14:1044.
14. Kraft SL, Gavin PR, Dehaan C, et al. Retrospective review of 50 canine intracranial tumors evaluated by magnetic resonance imaging. J Vet Intern Med 1997;11:218–25.
15. Graham JP, Newell SM, Voges AK, et al. The dural tail sign in the diagnosis of meningiomas. Vet Radiol Ultrasound 1998 Jul-Aug;39(4):297–302.
16. Hathcock JT. Low field magnetic resonance imaging characteristics of cranial vault meningiomas in 13 dogs. Vet Radiol Ultrasound 1996;37:257–63.
17. Bentley RT. Magnetic resonance imaging diagnosis of brain tumors in dogs. Vet J 2015 Aug;205(2):204–16.
18. Edwards MR, Garcia Mora JK, Fowler KM, et al. Magnetic resonance and computed tomographic imaging characteristics and potential molecular mechanisms of feline meningioma associated calvarial hyperostosis. Vet Comp Oncol 2024 Jun;22(2):174–85.
19. Nafe LA. Meningiomas in cats: A retrospective clinical study of 36 cases. J Am Vet Med Assoc 1979;174:1224–7.
20. Koestner A, Bilzer T, Fatzer R. Histological classification of tumors of the nervous system of domestic animals. In: Koestner A, Bilzer T, Fatzer R, editors. Histological classification of tumors of the nervous system of domestic animals WHO international classification of tumors of domestic animals5. Washington, DC, USA: Armed Forces Institute of Pathology; 1999. p. 22.
21. Fages J, Oura TJ, Sutherland-Smith J, et al. Atypical and malignant canine intracranial meningiomas may have lower apparent diffusion coefficient values than benign tumors. Vet Radiol Ultrasound 2020 Jan;61(1):40–7.
22. Wisner ER, Dickinson PJ, Higgins RJ. Magnetic resonance imaging features of canine intracranial neoplasia. Vet Radiol Ultrasound 2011;52:S52–61.
23. Mai W, Burke EE, Reetz JA, et al. High-field MRI using standard pulse sequences has moderate to substantial interobserver agreement and good accuracy for differentiation between intracranial extra-axial histiocytic sarcoma and meningioma in dogs. Vet Radiol Ultrasound 2022 Mar;63(2):176–84.
24. James FM, da Costa RC, Fauber A, et al. Clinical and MRI findings in three dogs with polycystic meningiomas. J Am Anim Hosp Assoc 2012 Sep-Oct;48(5):331–8.
25. McDonnell JJ, Kalbko K, Keating JH, et al. Multiple meningiomas in three dogs. J Am Anim Hosp Assoc 2007;43:201–8.

26. Tamura S, Tamura Y, Nakamoto Y, et al. MR imaging of histiocytic sarcoma of the canine brain. Vet Radiol Ultrasound 2009;50:178–81.
27. Thongtharb A, Uchida K, Chambers JK, et al. Histological and immunohisto-chemical studies on primary intracranial canine histiocytic sarcomas. J Vet Med Sci 2016;78:593–9.
28. Mariani CL, Jennings MK, Olby NJ, et al. Histiocytic sarcoma with central nervous system involvement in dogs: 19 cases (2006-2012). J Vet Intern Med 2015;29: 607–13.
29. Moore PF. A review of histiocytic diseases of dogs and cats. Veterinary Pathology 2014;51:167–84.
30. Wada M, Hasegawa D, Hamamoto Y, et al. Comparisons among MRI signs, apparent diffusion coefficient, and fractional anisotropy in dogs with a solitary intra-cranial meningioma or histiocytic sarcoma. Vet Radiol Ultrasound 2017;58:422–32.
31. Ishikawa C, Ito D, Kitagawa M, et al. Comparison of conventional magnetic reso-nance imaging and nonenhanced three dimensional time-of-flight magnetic reso-nance angiography findings between dogs with meningioma and dogs with intracranial histiocytic sarcoma: 19 cases (2010-2014). J Am Vet Med Assoc 2016;248:1139–47.
32. DeJesus A, Cohen EB, Galban E, et al. Magnetic resonance imaging features of intraventricular ependymomas in five cats. Vet Radiol Ultrasound 2017 May;58(3): 326–33.
33. Westworth DR, Dickinson PJ, Vernau W, et al. Choroid plexus tumors in 56 dogs (1985-2007). J Vet Intern Med 2008 Sep-Oct;22(5):1157–65.
34. Thomas WB, Wheeler SJ, Kramer R, et al. Magnetic resonance imaging features of primary brain tumors in dogs. Vet Radiol Ultrasound 1996;37:20–7.
35. Hecht S, Adams WH. MRI of brain disease in veterinary patients part 2: Acquired brain disorders. Vet Clin North Am Small Anim Pract 2010 Jan;40(1):39–63.
36. Vural SA, Besalti O, Ilhan F, et al. Ventricular ependymoma in a German Shepherd dog. Vet J 2006 Jul;172(1):185–7.
37. Young BD, Levine JM, Porter BF, et al. Magnetic resonance imaging features of intracranial astrocytomas and oligodendrogliomas in dogs. Vet Radiol Ultrasound 2011 Mar-Apr;52(2):132–41.
38. Jose-Lopez R, Gutierrez-Quintana R, de la Fuente C, et al. Clinical features, diag-nosis, and survival analysis of dogs with glioma. J Vet Intern Med 2021 Jul;35(4): 1902–17.
39. Bentley RT, Ober CP, Anderson KL, et al. Canine intracranial gliomas: relationship between magnetic resonance imaging criteria and tumor type and grade. Vet J 2013 Nov;198(2):463–71.
40. Koehler JW, Miller AD, Miller CR, et al. A Revised Diagnostic Classification of Canine Glioma: Towards Validation of the Canine Glioma Patient as a Naturally Occurring Preclinical Model for Human Glioma. J Neuropathol Exp Neurol 2018 Nov 1;77(11):1039–54.
41. Glamann S, Jeffery ND, Levine JM, et al. The "Claw Sign" may aid in axial local-ization in cases of peripherally located canine glioma on MRI. Vet Radiol Ultra-sound 2023 Jul;64(4):706–12.
42. Wolff CA, Holmes SP, Young BD, et al. Magnetic resonance imaging for the differ-entiation of neoplastic, inflammatory, and cerebrovascular brain disease in dogs. J Vet Intern Med 2012 May-Jun;26(3):589–97.
43. Cervera V, Mai W, Vite CH, et al. Comparative magnetic resonance imaging find-ings between gliomas and presumed cerebrovascular accidents in dogs. Vet Ra-diol Ultrasound 2011 Jan-Feb;52(1):33–40.

44. Sutherland-Smith J, King R, Faissler D, et al. Magnetic resonance imaging apparent diffusion coefficients for histologically confirmed intracranial lesions in dogs. Vet Radiol Ultrasound 2011 Mar-Apr;52(2):142–8.
45. Johnson PJ, Rivard BC, Wood JH, et al. Relationship between histological tumor margins and magnetic resonance imaging signal intensities in brain neoplasia of dogs. J Vet Intern Med 2022 May;36(3):1039–48.
46. Rossmeisl JH, Clapp K, Pancotto TE, et al. Canine Butterfly Glioblastomas: A Neuroradiological Review. Front Vet Sci 2016 May 19;3:40.
47. Schweizer-Gorgas D, Henke D, Oevermann A, et al. Magnetic resonance imaging features of canine gliomatosis cerebri. Vet Radiol Ultrasound 2018 Mar; 59(2):180–7.
48. Lipsitz D, Higgins RJ, Kortz GD, et al. Glioblastoma multiforme: Clinical findings, magnetic resonance imaging, and pathology in five dogs. Vet Pathol 2003;40: 659–69.
49. Giri DK, Aloisio F, Ajithdoss DK, et al. Giant cell glioblastoma in the cerebrum of a Pembroke welsh corgi. J Comp Pathol 2011;144:324–7.
50. Wolf M, PedroiaV Higgins RJ, Koblik PD, et al. Intracranial ring enhancing lesions in dogs: a correlative CT scanning and neuropathologic study. Vet Radiol Ultrasound 1995;36:16–20.
51. Kelly PJ, Daumas-Duport C, Scheithauer BW, et al. Stereotactic histologic correlations of computed tomography- and magnetic resonance imaging-defined abnormalities in patients with glial neoplasms. Mayo Clin Proc 1987;62:450–9.
52. Kelly PJ, Daumas-Duport C, Kispert DB, et al. Imaging-based stereotaxic serial biopsies in untreated intracranial glial neoplasms. J Neurosurg 1987;66:865–74.
53. Watanabe M, Tanaka R, Takeda N. Magnetic resonance imaging and histopathology of cerebral gliomas. Neuroradiology 1992;34(6):463–9.
54. Garcia-Mora J, Parker RL, Cecere T, et al. The T2-FLAIR mismatch sign as an imaging biomarker for oligodendrogliomas in dogs. J Vet Intern Med 2023 Jul-Aug; 37(4):1447–54.
55. Gruber A, Leschnik M, Kneissl S, et al. Gliomatosis cerebri in a dog. J Vet Med A Physiol Pathol Clin Med 2006;53(8):435–8.
56. Liatis T, Hammond G, Chapman GE, et al. MRI findings in a young dog with gliomatosis cerebri. J Small Anim Pract 2022 Jan;63(1):83.
57. Porter B, de Lahunta A, Summers B. Gliomatosis cerebri in six dogs. Vet Pathol 2003 Jan;40(1):97–102.
58. Rodenas S, Pumarola M, Gaitero L, et al. Magnetic resonance imaging findings in 40 dogs with histologically confirmed intracranial tumours. Vet J 2011;187(1): 85–91.
59. Fukuoka H, Sasaki J, Kamishina H, et al. Gliomatosis Cerebelli in a Saint Bernard Dog. J Comp Pathol 2012;147:37–41.
60. Martin-Vaquero P, da Costa RC, Wolk KE, et al. MRI features of gliomatosis cerebri in a dog. Vet Radiol Ultrasound 2012;53:189–92.
61. Canal S, Bernardini M, Pavone S, et al. Primary diffuse leptomeningeal gliomatosis in 2 dogs. Can Vet J 2013;54:1075–9.
62. Carrera I, Richter H, Beckmann K, et al. Evaluation of intracranial neoplasia and noninfectious meningoencephalitis in dogs by use of short echo time, single voxel proton magnetic resonance spectroscopy at 3.0 Tesla. Am J Vet Res 2016 May;77(5):452–62.
63. Stadler KL, Ober CP, Feeney DA, et al. Multivoxel proton magnetic resonance spectroscopy of inflammatory and neoplastic lesions of the canine brain at 3.0 T. Am J Vet Res 2014 Nov;75(11):982–9.

64. Dowling C, Bollen AW, Noworolski SM, et al. Preoperative proton MR spectroscopic imaging of brain tumors: correlation with histopathologic analysis of resection specimens. Am J Neuroradiol 2001;22:604–12.

65. Peng SL, Chen CF, Liu HJ, et al. Analysis of parametric histogram from dynamic contrast-enhanced MRI: application in evaluating brain tumor response to radiotherapy. NMR Biomed 2012;26:443–50.

66. Hirai T, Murakami R, Nakamura H, et al. Prognostic value of perfusion MR imaging of high-grade astrocytomas: long-term follow-up study. AJNR Am J Neuroradiol 2008;29:1505–10.

67. Law M, Young RJ, Babb JS, et al. Gliomas: predicting time to progression or survival with cerebral blood volume measurements at dynamic susceptibility-weighted contrast-enhanced perfusion MR imaging. Radiology 2008;247:490–8.

68. MacLeod AG, Dickinson PJ, LeCouteur RA, et al. Quantitative assessment of blood volume and permeability in cerebral mass lesions using dynamic contrast-enhanced computed tomography in the dog. Acad Radiol 2009;16: 1187–95.

69. Zhao Q, Lee S, Kent M, et al. Dynamic contrast-enhanced magnetic resonance imaging of canine brain tumors. Vet Radiol Ultrasound 2010;51:122–9.

70. Chenevert TL, Sundgren PC, Ross BD. Diffusion imaging: insight to cell status and cytoarchitecture. Neuroimaging Clin N Am 2006;16:619–32.

71. Chenevert TL, Stegman LD, Taylor JM, et al. Diffusion magnetic resonance imaging: an early surrogate marker of therapeutic efficacy in brain tumors. J Natl Cancer Inst 2000;92(24):2029–36.

72. Lee SK. Diffusion tensor and perfusion imaging of brain tumors in high-field MR imaging. Neuroimaging Clin N Am 2012;22:123–34.

73. Romani R, Tang WJ, Mao Y, et al. Diffusion tensor magnetic resonance imaging for predicting the consistency of intracranial meningiomas. Acta Neurochir 2014;156:1837–45.

74. Dickinson PJ. Advances in diagnostic and treatment modalities for intracranial tumors. J Vet Intern Med 2014 Jul-Aug;28(4):1165–85.

75. Wada M, Hasegawa D, Hamamoto Y, et al. Comparison of Canine and Feline Meningiomas Using the Apparent Diffusion Coefficient and Fractional Anisotropy. Front Vet Sci 2021 Jan 11;7:614026.

76. Nandu H, Wen PY, Huang RY. Imaging in neuro-oncology. Ther Adv Neurol Disord 2018 28;11:1756286418759865.

77. Segtnan EA, Hess S, Grupe P, et al. ^{18}F-fluorodeoxyglucose PET/computed tomography for primary brain tumors. Pet Clin 2015 Jan;10(1):59–73.

78. Purandare NC, Puranik A, Shah S, et al. Common malignant brain tumors: can 18F-FDG PET/CT aid in differentiation? Nucl Med Commun 2017 Dec;38(12):1109–16.

79. Herholz K, Coope D, Jackson A. Metabolic and molecular imaging in neuro-oncology. Lancet Neurol 2007 Aug;6(8):711–24.

80. Das K, Mittal B, Vasistha R, et al. Role of (18)F-fluorodeoxyglucose Positron Emission Tomography scan in differentiating enhancing brain tumors. Indian J Nucl Med 2011;26(4):171–6.

81. Takahashi M, Soma T, Mukasa A, et al. Pattern of FDG and MET Distribution in High- and Low-Grade Gliomas on PET Images. Clin Nucl Med 2019 Apr;44(4): 265–71.

82. Delbeke D, Meyerowitz C, Lapidus RL, et al. Optimal cutoff levels of F-18 fluorodeoxyglucose uptake in the differentiation of low-grade from high-grade brain tumors with PET. Radiology 1995 Apr;195(1):47–52.

83. Jacobs AH, Thomas A, Kracht LW, et al. 18F-fluoro-l-thymidine and 11C-methyl-methionine as markers of increased transport and proliferation in brain tumors. J Nucl Med 2005;46:1948–58.

84. Chen W, Cloughesy T, Kamdar N, et al. Imaging proliferation in brain tumors with 18F-FLT PET: comparison with 18F-FDG. J Nucl Med 2005;46:945–52.

85. Hutterer M, Nowosielski M, Putzer D, et al. [18F]-fluoro-ethyl-L-tyrosine PET: a valuable diagnostic tool in neuro-oncology, but not all that glitters is glioma. Neuro Oncol 2013;3:341–51.

86. Kang BT, Son YD, Lee SR, et al. FDG uptake of normal canine brain assessed by high-resolution research tomography-positron emission tomography and 7 T-magnetic resonance imaging. J Vet Med Sci 2012 Oct;74(10):1261–7.

87. Lee MS, Ko J, Lee AR, et al. Effects of anesthetic protocol on normal canine brain uptake of 18F-FDG assessed by PET/CT. Vet Radiol Ultrasound 2010 Mar-Apr; 51(2):130–5.

88. Irimajiri M, Miller MA, Green MA, et al. Cerebral metabolism in dogs assessed by (18)F-FDG PET: a pilot study to understand physiological changes in behavioral disorders in dogs. J Vet Med Sci 2010 Jan;72(1):1–6.

89. Kang BT, Kim SG, Lim CY, et al. Correlation between fluorodeoxyglucose positron emission tomography and magnetic resonance imaging findings of non-suppurative meningoencephalitis in 5 dogs. Can Vet J 2010 Sep;51(9):986–92.

90. Eom KD, Lim CY, Gu SH, et al. Positron emission tomography features of canine necrotizing meningoencephalitis. Vet Radiol Ultrasound 2008 Nov-Dec;49(6): 595–9.

91. Brennan KM, Roos MS, Budinger TF, et al. A study of radiation necrosis and edema in the canine brain using positron emission tomography and magnetic resonance imaging. Radiat Res 1993 Apr;134(1):43–53.

92. Jones K, Loeber S, Cameron S, et al. 18F- Fluorodeoxyglucose positron emission tomography/magnetic resonance imaging in canine brain tumor patients: a pilot study. International veterinary radiologists association European veterinary diagnostic imaging joint scientific conference. University College Dublin, Dublin, Ireland. June 18-23, 2023. Abstract presented in poster format.

93. Kang BT, Park C, Yoo JH, et al. 18F-fluorodeoxyglucose positron emission tomography and magnetic resonance imaging findings of primary intracranial histiocytic sarcoma in a dog. J Vet Med Sci 2009 Oct;71(10):1397–401.

94. Yun T, Koo Y, Kim S, et al. Characteristics of ^{18}F-FDG and ^{18}F-FDOPA PET in an 8-year-old neutered male Yorkshire Terrier dog with glioma: long-term chemotherapy using hydroxyurea plus imatinib with prednisolone and immunoreactivity for PDGFR-β and LAT1. Vet Q 2021;41(1):163–71.

95. Banzato T, Bernardini M, Cherubini GB, et al. Texture analysis of magnetic resonance images to predict histologic grade of meningiomas in dogs. Am J Vet Res 2017 Oct;78(10):1156–62.

96. Banzato T, Bernardini M, Cherubini GB, et al. A methodological approach for deep learning to distinguish between meningiomas and gliomas on canine MR-images. BMC Vet Res 2018 Oct 22;14(1):317.

97. Wanamaker MW, Vernau KM, Taylor SL, et al. Classification of neoplastic and inflammatory brain disease using MRI texture analysis in 119 dogs. Vet Radiol Ultrasound 2021 Jul;62(4):445–54.

98. Barge P, Oevermann A, Maiolini A, et al. Machine learning predicts histologic type and grade of canine gliomas based on MRI texture analysis. Vet Radiol Ultrasound 2023 Jul;64(4):724–32.

Biopsy of Brain Lesions

Nick D. Jeffery, BVSc, PhD, MSc, FRCVS

KEYWORDS

- Histopathology • Diagnosis • Accuracy • Dog • Intracranial

KEY POINTS

- Tissue or cytology specimens are necessary for accurate diagnosis of intracranial lesions.
- Brain biopsy is generally safe and provides accurate information about sampled lesions.
- Three-dimensional-printed guides are customizable and reduce costs.

INTRODUCTION

In medicine, generally, establishing a specific diagnosis is a key step in ensuring that appropriate treatment is selected and, ideally, this principle should not be abandoned when treating diseases of the brain. However, brain disease presents several obstacles to straightforward diagnosis in many cases, especially in veterinary medicine. First, the brain is relatively inaccessible for many tests (apart from imaging) because of its enclosure in the skull and separation from the circulation by the blood-brain barrier. Second, there is a widespread perception that directs biopsy of the brain is risky for the patient and so is often avoided. Third, it can be costly to obtain direct biopsies and the increase in cost can be prohibitive for pet owners who are already stretched financially by expensive imaging diagnostics. Lastly, there is a strong cognitive bias in veterinary medicine that obtaining a comprehensive tissue diagnosis may not alter the way many brain lesions—especially tumors—are treated, because there currently are not well-defined specifically-targeted treatment pathways. As a consequence of these effects, it is common that brain diseases in animals are incompletely diagnosed.

Brain lesions are almost exclusively initially recognized on computed tomography (CT) or MRI and many lesions have characteristic appearance[1,2] that tends to militate against biopsy because it may be considered that it would expose the animal to risk without benefit. On the other hand, one of the key diagnostic definitions is to distinguish between classes of disease, such as between inflammatory or infectious (often fungal) and neoplastic lesions because they may often look very similar (**Fig. 1**). The second reason for biopsy is to be able to classify a neoplasm because it may be of benefit in making treatment decisions.

Department of Small Animal Clinical Sciences, College of Veterinary Medicine and Biomedical Sciences, Texas A&M University, TX, USA
E-mail address: njeffery@cvm.tamu.edu

Vet Clin Small Anim 55 (2025) 41–55
https://doi.org/10.1016/j.cvsm.2024.07.005   vetsmall.theclinics.com

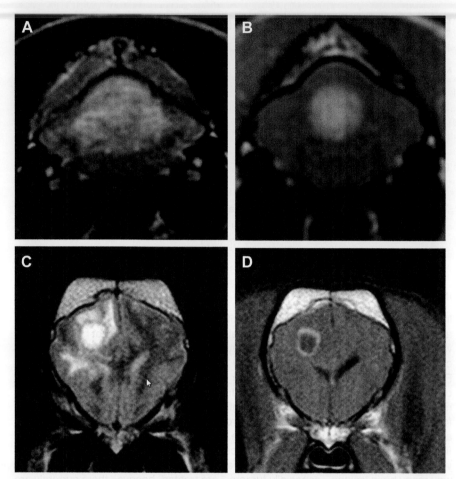

Fig. 1. Examples of magnetic resonance images in which the final diagnosis is unexpected. (*A* and *B*) T2-weighted and contrast-enhanced T1-weighted images of the cerebellum of a cat. The histopathologic diagnosis was aspergillosis.(*C* and *D*) T2-weighted and contrast-enhanced T1-weighted images of the cerebral frontal lobes of a 5-year-old French bulldog. The histologic diagnosis was necrotizing leukoencephalitis. (Images courtesy of Dr. Thomas Flegel and Dr. Sarah Gutmann, University of Leipzig, Germany. C & D published earlier in Flegel T (2017) Breed-Specific Magnetic Resonance Imaging Characteristics of Necrotizing Encephalitis in Dogs. Front. Vet. Sci. 4:203. https://doi.org/10.3389/fvets.2017.00203.).

ALTERNATIVES TO BIOPSY

For the most part, diagnosis of brain lesions in dogs and cats leans heavily on imaging, where their characteristics are used to make an informed guess. However, diagnostic tests must be extremely reliable and accurate to be useful in clinical medicine. The important analysis of diagnostic testing is defining sensitivity and specificity and these need to be in the high 90% range to be appropriately reliable.

Are Images Sufficient?

Assumed image-based diagnoses are insufficiently accurate in many cases in humans; Yan and colleagues (2016)[3] reported a sensitivity of 72% to 91% and a positive predictive value of 92% to 95% (in a sample containing 13% non-tumor diag-noses). Thus, although the imaging-based diagnosis of a specific brain tumor is certainly quite likely to be accurate, there is a substantial proportion of misdiagnosis, which may be detrimental for those patients. In veterinary medicine, several studies concur that agreement between observers and between MRI diagnosis and histopath-ological diagnosis may be inadequate for reliable clinical diagnosis and treatment allo-cation.[4] Even sophisticated imaging methods, such as diffusion-weighted MRI or texture analysis, fail at too high a rate to replace histologic diagnosis.[5,6] Similarly, although magnetic resonance spectroscopy (MRS) has a high accuracy, available data suggest that the categorizations are insufficiently reliable for clinical diagnosis in dogs.[7]

Cerebrospinal Fluid Analysis

Cerebrospinal fluid (CSF) analysis is a well-established method of detecting disease in the central nervous system and most suspected autoimmune inflammatory lesions in humans and animals are presumptively diagnosed on imaging and CSF analysis without further attempts at biopsy (although there are some inflammatory lesions that do not appear to be associated with increased CSF cell count).[8] CSF analysis can reveal non-specific signs of inflammation and potentially also detect infectious organisms, such as bacteria[9] and fungi (most commonly cryptococcus[10,11]). Unfortunately, few tu-mors appear to exfoliate sufficient numbers of cells for CSF to be diagnostic, although choroid plexus tumors may be an exception: in a study $\sim$50% of samples from dogs with choroid plexus carcinomas were reported to have neoplastic cells in the CSF.[12] Cells diagnostic for histiocytic sarcoma have also been detected in CSF.[13,14]

In contrast, for the most common brain tumors in dogs (meningioma and glioma), CSF reveals, at best, non-specific alterations such as mild increase in cell counts in some individuals[15,16] but neoplastic cells are not detected on routine cytologic examination.

Systemic Investigations

It is sometimes possible to surmise indirectly that an intracranial lesion is caused by infectious disease if infectious disease is located elsewhere in the body, especially the thorax or lymph nodes. For example, a brain lesion may be associated with an intrathoracic fungal granuloma, or perhaps associated with discospondylitis or a uri-nary tract infection. Similar educated guesses about a brain mass may also be possible with thoracic masses diagnosed as neoplastic and of a type that is likely to metastasize to the brain (or elsewhere), such as hemangiosarcoma or mammary tumor.

Blood analysis will sometimes give clues to the cause of a brain lesion, such as serum or urine galactomannan antigen testing if aspergillosis (or other fungal lesions) is suspected, or thrombocytopenia associated with intracranial hemorrhage.

WHAT INFORMATION IS REQUIRED FROM A BRAIN BIOPSY?

After exhausting alternative indirect methods, many questions often remain about lesion diagnosis. There are 2 levels of information from brain biopsy that are currently needed in veterinary medicine: (i) What class of disease is the lesion? (ii) What is the subtype or grade of disease?

Differentiating a non-neoplastic from a neoplastic lesion is clearly important because of the contrasting treatment recommendations. The need for differentiation of various types of neoplastic lesions in veterinary medicine might currently be questioned because they are often treated similarly (by radiotherapy). On the other hand, to make therapeutic progress, there is a need to be more certain about diagnosis and then retrospective review of case series could aid in determining whether different treatments lead to different outcomes within specific diagnostic categories. Nowadays, the classification of human brain tumors relies upon a series of tests that depend not only on histology but also require genetic analysis, which implies that biopsy is currently essential.[17] Dog brain tumor classification is not at such an advanced stage but the poor agreement between pathologist assessment of histologic type and grade[18] suggests the need for this type of analysis in the future to enable more precisely targeted treatments.

An alternative viewpoint is that pragmatic treatment trials do not necessarily demand such highly specific diagnosis because lesions can simply be categorized on imaging features alone and outcome determined for that defined category (even though the diagnosis within an imaging-defined category might be varied).

HOW TO TAKE A BRAIN BIOPSY

The most obvious biopsy method is open surgery, but there are many drawbacks and so less invasive methods are usually preferred. One unique problem with acquiring a brain biopsy that is not commonly problematic for biopsy of other organs is the movement of the brain that can occur when the skull (and particularly the dura mater) is opened.[19] When the limiting structures are opened, the brain will move and the relative position of the internal structures, including the target lesion, will alter and previously identified landmarks may not be reliable guides to the target. This brain movement will not be sufficient to cause problems when taking a biopsy of a large lesion but might be for those of only a few millimeters. In human medicine, it is also recognized that different locations within a single glioma may contain different types of tumor cell as defined by genetic or chromosomal changes,[20] so precise targeting (and obtaining multiple biopsies) is important for accurate diagnosis.

Open Biopsy

Open biopsy is a straightforward option for brain biopsy because it requires few specialized items of equipment, only the instruments required to open the skull and dura. The most common reason for open biopsy will be its availability during definitive tumor removal. This type of biopsy procedure is for confirmation of diagnosis rather than to guide intra-operative or post-operative decision-making.

An alternative approach during open surgery is to use biopsies to guide the invasiveness of a procedure. Sometimes, it is not known what type of lesion is being approached and it can be useful to take small samples following first exposure of the lesion in an attempt to make a more precise diagnosis during the surgery. For instance, initially the question to the attending pathologist might be "Is this neoplastic or inflammatory?" but then a later question might be "Is it possible to identify a pathogen?" or "What type of tumor do you think it is?" Squash smear techniques can be highly reliable in distinguishing between infections and tumors as a first important classification.[21] Moreover, although frozen section histology is often used for intraoperative diagnosis in human medicine, intraoperative cytology provides comparably reliable diagnoses[22] and is readily available in the more limited resource environments that apply in veterinary medicine. Veterinary experience with intraoperative brain cytology is also highly supportive of its reliability.[23–25]

The appearance of a brain mass during surgery may be quite variable. Those that may be found in the subarachnoid space (predominantly meningioma but also including histiocytic sarcoma, lymphoma, and infectious granuloma) are usually easily recognized and biopsied. In contrast, mass lesions within the brain parenchyma (predominantly glial tumors but also including granulomas, lymphoma, and hematomas) may not have clear margins and it may be difficult to detect the lesion with the naked eye. Notably, gliomas are often almost indistinguishable from normal brain tissue in surgery. Fluorescence-guided surgery, in which a fluorescent agent is injected intravenously, provides a potential means of circumventing this problem because these agents accumulate in regions of impaired blood-brain barrier function. Unfortunately, although fluorescent agents can be useful in many specific cases, they may not be so reliable in low-grade tumors.[26,27] Intraoperative guidance using ultrasound provides an alternative method to increase precision in obtaining tissue from a target deep in the brain during open surgery.[28] Intraoperative ultrasound is not commonly described in veterinary neurosurgery, but a recent report described how freeze-core biopsies obtained under ultrasound guidance might provide useful specimens.[29]

A key component of intra-operative cytology or histology interpretation is effective and direct communication both before and during the procedure with the pathologist reading the biopsy material.[30] The most important aspect is for both partners to understand what decisions are required at each stage. For instance, from the surgeon's point of view, the question is often whether more surgery would likely be beneficial or whether the pathologist's diagnosis would suggest that alternative therapies, such as anti-microbial medications, may be more appropriate. Direct live conversation may also be necessary to ascertain the pathologist's confidence in the diagnosis so that the option of obtaining further specimens can be considered. The benefit of this type of iterative diagnostic process is that the surgery can be limited to what is required to formulate a treatment plan (which may include attempted total excision) and no more.

A notable advantage of open biopsy is that it usually allows biopsy-created hemorrhage to be clearly seen and appropriately treated. Numerous hemostatic agents can be applied at open surgery, including bipolar diathermy, Gelfoam, and surgical cellulose. A major disadvantage of open biopsy is that is necessitates preparation like that required for a definitive surgical procedure and so entails considerable cost, which is often a deterrent for owners.

Freehand Image-Guided Biopsy

Many brain lesions in dogs are large (several centimeters in diameter) and so freehand biopsy through a burr hole would appear likely to successfully obtain a diagnostic biopsy. On the other hand, such large lesions might often be less likely to be considered targets for biopsy because their nature is often more likely to be strongly presumed, although still susceptible to error.[4] Freehand biopsy has largely been supplanted by the availability of more sophisticated techniques, although the success rate for obtaining diagnostic biopsies in a series was reportedly high (94%).[31]

Stereotactic Frame-Based Biopsy

Stereotactic devices, inside which the skull is rigidly held in place by ear bars,[32] have been used for decades in neuroscience research to guide injections into very specific sites in the brain, by reference to external landmarks on the skull (notably "bregma"—the suture where the 2 frontal and 2 parietal bones meet). This same technique, using commercially available or modified devices, has been used in veterinary medicine for brain biopsy, by mounting a biopsy needle into the stereotactic holder. Typical devices for brain biopsy include Trucut needles and side-cutting 16G needles (**Fig. 2**).[33] Initial investigation on a commercially available device suggested high accuracy (~1 mm

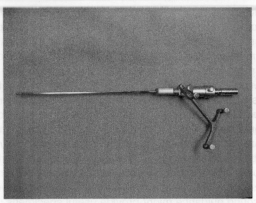

Fig. 2. Sedan side-cutting brain biopsy needle inside the stereotactic needle guide sleeve, to which are attached some reflective markers for navigation. (Images courtesy of Dr. Thomas Flegel and Dr. Sarah Gutmann, University of Leipzig, Germany.).

deviations from target) in needle placement in cadavers.[34] High (~95%) success rates in biopsy and diagnostic accuracy were also found in analyzing biopsy obtained via a modified commercial device,[35] a novel device designed especially for veterinary patients,[36] and an MRI-compatible frame-based device.[33,37]

When using this type of instrument, measurements from the skull surface and in reference to recognizable landmarks (such as the sagittal crest) are determined from cross-sectional images (usually MRI, but sometimes CT) to enable the biopsy instrument to reach the lesion. The animal is then positioned in the stereotactic device and secured, usually using ear bars placed into the external auditory meatus. The appropriate area of the skull is exposed through open surgery and the needle holder is positioned over the skull surface. A burr hole is made at the designated site, the dura cauterized and cut to allow unimpeded needle penetration, and the biopsy needle inserted. Several samples are taken from the lesion where possible, especially at the margins and superficial and deep layers.

The advantages of this system are its availability, relatively low cost (compared to other systems—see later), and ease of use. Drawbacks can be the bulkiness and difficulty in working around the device while it is in place (it can be difficult to reach the skull surface around the [often non-sterile] device during surgery) and, in some devices, the limited flexibility in how the needle can be positioned (older devices only allow control of needle position in the 3 orthogonal planes without possible arc-derived access). Devices that are only CT-compatible have the drawback that many lesions are not well delineated on CT, as compared to MRI.

Other Frame-Based Biopsy

A stereotactic device designed for use in human breast biopsy[38] and a simple mechanical vector targeting device,[39] which both use an angled guide to denote a grid that designates the biopsy trajectory, have also been investigated. Both devices had a high success rate in reaching their targets and, in a series, obtaining high-quality biopsies.[39]

Stereotactic Biopsy by Neuronavigation

The advent of infra-red motion capture systems has allowed the development of frameless biopsy. In this context, "frameless" is used to refer to the absence of a stereotactic frame to calculate the site of entry and biopsy needle trajectory. The advantage of these systems is that after MR images and real-life anatomy have been co-registered, it is possible to "see" what areas of the brain can be reached using a device inserted at a specific site and trajectory and to see the effects of small adjustments in position. These systems allow precisely targeted biopsy, even from small lesions (after mounting the biopsy instrument on a frame for stability). Although a CT-guided system is available,[40] because MRI is used more commonly for diagnosing brain lesions in dogs, the most widely used frameless system in veterinary medicine is the MRI-compatible "Brainsight."[41]

Brainsight technique relies on "fiducial markers" that can be reproducibly attached to the head through mouthpieces and moldable dental material and their relationship with structures inside the cranium can be determined from MR images (**Fig. 3**). Once the MR images are uploaded to the computer system, the position of each fiducial marker is registered using the subject tracker (pointer device) and images acquired

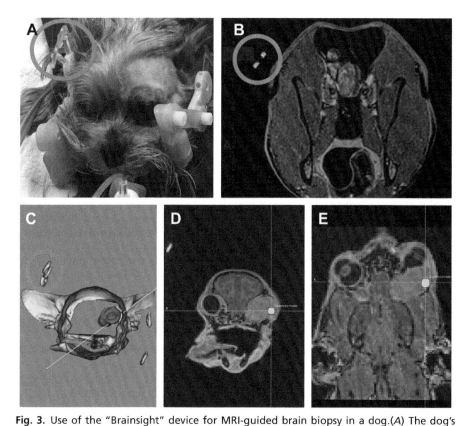

Fig. 3. Use of the "Brainsight" device for MRI-guided brain biopsy in a dog.(A) The dog's head is secured in a reproducible position using a bite plate (visible as a blue material close to the endotracheal tube). The bite plate is attached to a head frame system that includes "fiducial markers" (orange circle).(B) The fiducial markers (orange circle) are also visible on MRI thereby defining the position of the brain relative to the markers in both "real-life" and on images.(C) Composite reconstructed image showing a relationship between fiducial markers (1 set highlighted with orange circle) and the target lesion (magenta). The planned biopsy needle trajectory is shown in green.(D, E) Transverse and dorsal plane composite magnetic resonance images showing biopsy target site in the lesion (brown). (Images courtesy of Dr. Amanda Taylor, Southeast Veterinary Neurology, Virginia Beach, VA).

in conjunction with an optical position sensor. After registering the correspondence between MRI and real-life anatomy, the trajectories of biopsy needles through the brain can be planned. During the biopsy procedure, the head must be kept rigidly in place relative to the biopsy instrument, which is achieved with a head clamp and bars that can be screwed tightly against the skull.

A burr hole is then made in the skull and the biopsy needle inserted through an instrument sleeve held in an articulated arm attached to the head clamp. Usually, trajectories are made through the cerebral cortex because it is relatively safe to make a hole through this region without lasting deficits and large blood vessels can usually be avoided. Trajectories through the brainstem are used in human medicine[e.g.42] but are rarely, if ever, attempted in veterinary medicine. Tests on this system determined a mean placement error of 1.8 mm with an upper error bound of 3.3 mm, suggesting that lesions as small as 3.3 mm might be successfully biopsied with this system.[41] A similar device that has no frame at all was reported to successfully acquire diagnostic biopsies in 9/10 dogs.[43]

The advantages of this technique are the minimal invasiveness and precision (although this may be compromised by brain shift unless another scan is obtained after skull opening). The drawback is the cost of the equipment and the (prolonged) time required to set up the system for taking the biopsy.

Three-dimensional-Printed Biopsy Guides

Because of the high cost of computer-aided navigational biopsy, various alternative methods of guiding biopsy needles to the correct location have been investigated in veterinary medicine. The wide availability of 3-dimensional (3D)-printed guides has recently made this an attractive option with high reported rates of successful biopsy.

There are several ways to use 3D-printing to guide brain biopsy. One method incorporates screws placed into prominent bony landmarks that can then be used as the anchor points for the feet of a 3D-printed device that contains custom columns through which drill sleeves can be placed to guide making the burr hole and the biopsy needle sleeve can be placed to guide biopsy needle placement (**Fig. 4**).[44] The precision of this method was reported to be extremely high when tested in cadavers,[45] and yielded diagnostic biopsies in live patients.[46]

A second method is more like 3D-printed guides used elsewhere for orthopedic and spinal fixation systems, in which the guide plate is contoured to the skull surface based on CT or MR images.[47] This type of guide depends for accuracy on finding a unique foot area where they fit so that the sleeve hole will guide the drill and biopsy instrument exactly to the target. This can be problematic on the skull because it has few specific features, although using a large footplate will enhance the ability to match the exact contour of an individual skull. Perhaps, because of this difficulty and that of maintaining the correct positioning during drilling, the accuracy of this technique is less than that of some other stereotactic biopsy methods (with a biopsy needle placement error of 2–3 mm). There is a need to remove all soft tissue before placing such devices in contact with the skullbecause any slight deviation from precise placement will amplify the risk of missing the target.

A third method relies upon producing a 3D-printed mask that is contoured to fit precisely over the animal's face and nose, with an incorporated biopsy sleeve that will guide a biopsy device to the target lesion.[48] An obvious potential drawback of this type of mold is whether it will fit snugly enough to direct the biopsy but, although the targeting precision of this type of device has not been investigated, successful biopsy was reported in 5 of 5 clinical patients.

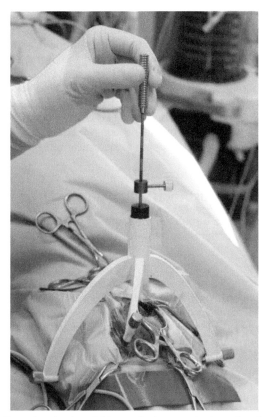

Fig. 4. Custom 3-dimensional printed biopsy device attached to the skull through screws inserted into zygomatic arches. The biopsy device is being inserted to reach the target. (Images courtesy of Dr. Thomas Flegel and Dr. Sarah Gutmann, University of Leipzig, Germany.).

Advantages to 3D-printed guides are the minimal invasiveness and low cost (compared with computer imaging). The low cost has also led to their use in human medicine in low- resource settings.[49] Disadvantages include the relative imprecision.

COMPLICATIONS OF BRAIN BIOPSY

There are many possible complications of brain biopsy that can be caused by inadvertent damage to intracranial structures, but one of the most common is failure to obtain a diagnostic sample. It has been estimated that ∼10% of brain biopsies obtained in humans are non-diagnostic[50] and a similar proportion has been reported in, albeit much smaller, veterinary populations.[33–37,43,46,48,51] The problems of failure to obtain a diagnostic sample can be attributed to the biopsy system itself (how accurately does it target the lesion?), the lesion itself (eg, a blood clot will not produce a reliably diagnostic biopsy sample), pathologist inexperience (not many veterinary pathologists are experienced in examining cytology specimens from brain biopsy), brain displacement upon opening the dura, or taking biopsies from inappropriate regions of the lesion. Methods to ameliorate most of these problems are obvious although it is difficult to mitigate the inaccuracies associated with brain displacement associated with dural opening. This problem can be solved with intraoperative MRI, although implying additional expense. However, brain lesions in small animals are frequently large and so minor brain displacement may not incur a great risk of mistargeting.

The most feared complications of brain biopsy are iatrogenic neural injury and hemorrhage. In most series of brain biopsies in humans, the overall complication rate is quite high ($\sim$25%)[52] but few of these complications are symptomatic and fewer still are associated with long-lasting neurologic deficits (0.5%) or biopsy-related death (0.8%). Available data suggest that it is uncommon (0/62 patients) to require re-operation to attend to post-biopsy bleeding in humans.[53] Complication rates in veterinary medicine are more difficult to quantify accurately because the case series report much smaller patient numbers but appear to be similar both overall and in terms of their impact on the animal.[33,35,36,51]

WHY DON'T VETERINARY NEUROLOGISTS TAKE MORE BRAIN BIOPSIES?

Stereotactic brain biopsy is a routine procedure in human medicine but is not often carried out in veterinary patients, for many possible reasons.

Expense

Diagnosis and management of intracranial lesions is expensive and unaffordable for many dog and cat owners. Even for those with sufficient funds available, it may prove difficult for a veterinary neurologist to persuade them that an additional expensive procedure is worthwhile. To some extent, this line of decision-making is tied up with potential risks and benefits (see below), and many owners would wish to see a clear benefit in terms of better treatment and survival if they are spending an additional few thousand dollars.

The costs of biopsy derive mainly from time under anesthesia and the capital cost of the necessary equipment. This cost can therefore be reduced by using cheap equipment that requires little time under anesthesia, such as 3D-printed guides. Although some of these may be slightly less accurate than more sophisticated systems, the trade-off in terms of enhanced diagnosis at low cost might be beneficial overall.

Fear of Injury

When contemplating treatment for an intracranial lesion (usually a brain tumor), there is an understandable concern to avoid exacerbating the clinical signs and, whereas treatment-related complications are easy to justify, complications related to an equivocally useful diagnostic procedure may be difficult for owners to accept. However, as demonstrated in the discussion earlier, serious and long-lasting complications from brain biopsy are rare and so perhaps should not be strongly weighted in discussion with pet owners.

Concern About Missed Diagnosis

Similar to concerns about possible injury, it can be worrying as a veterinarian to recommend an expensive test that turns out not to be diagnostic, and this might account for a reluctance to pursue brain biopsy in some cases. Again, the data that are available from both human and veterinary sources suggest that brain biopsy has a high ($\sim$95% agreement with surgical or necropsy specimens) diagnostic rate and routinely provides specific diagnoses.[37,54]

Owner Resistance to Procedures on the Brain

Many owners react with alarm to the possibility of their pet having procedures carried out on the brain, perhaps sometimes because of almost superstitious beliefs about the possible outcomes. As a result, many owners, even those with sufficient funds, are unwilling to go ahead with definitive treatments, such as surgery or radiotherapy for brain tumors, even though post-treatment survival is often prolonged.[55]

This reluctance to engage with treatment of brain lesions may deter owners from pursuing biopsy, but alternatively it could be considered that the "halfway house" of taking a biopsy to confirm a diagnosis may encourage owners to go ahead with definitive therapies.

Veterinary Concern that the Outcome of Biopsy Will Not Change What We Do Afterward

Veterinary neurologists and oncologists commonly will consider that a lesion that is visible on a scan can be treated by the same therapy without needing to know a specific diagnosis. For instance, in veterinary medicine, it is often argued that any brain tumor (and even some inflammatory lesions)[56] can be effectively treated with radiotherapy and so why would biopsy be useful? However, this leads to a problem that is insoluble without brain biopsy: we do not know the best treatment for a specific lesion because we do not know what it is, and we don't know what it is because we often think that the biopsy won't make a difference and so we do not take one. Of course, without biopsy there is also the possibility of erroneous diagnosis.

In dealing with brain neoplasia in particular, the experience in human medicine is that by obtaining a specific diagnosis a specific treatment can be recommended. It would be expected that the same would be true in animals, but such an outcome would be dependent on obtaining outcome data and histologic specimens from many hundreds or thousands of cases. The question of whether the eventual outcome in terms of enhanced, but more costly, therapy would be supported by owners must also be considered: would the expense entailed in biopsy and subsequent specific therapies be affordable and practical for a large enough proportion of pet owners?

The question of whether to obtain a brain biopsy in a small animal patient becomes most pressing when dealing with a patient in which there is considerable doubt over the diagnosis and direction of subsequent therapy and that is owned by someone who can afford intensive therapy. The most common questions are in deciding whether a lesion may be inflammatory or neoplastic or, alternatively, distinguishing between glioma and hematoma, both of which may be uncertain from images alone. In human medicine, not only is there a strong rationale for biopsy of suspected neoplastic lesions in the brain because of the link to specific treatments from specific diagnoses but brain biopsy can also have a major impact on treatment decisions in non-neoplastic diseases.[57]

FUTURE OPTIONS

In human medicine, more detailed and precise methods for taking biopsies, such as robotics and augmented reality are beginning to enter the clinic[58] although, considering the expense involved, it would appear unlikely that these options will transfer to veterinary medicine, in the near future at least. Alternative methods to obtain biopsy information, such as "liquid biopsy" have been intensely investigated in humans[59] and undergone preliminary investigation in animals.[60,61] Liquid biopsy material has great promise because there is potentially so much information available, including the potential to analyze RNA, DNA, proteins, and lipids circulating in both CSF and serum. However, there are many steps between detecting possible markers associated with specific tumors and using that as a diagnostic test that is sufficiently reliable to direct treatment plans. Furthermore, during the development stage, it is essential that histologic material is available to correlate the content of liquid biopsy with histologic diagnosis. Currently, this diagnostic method shows promise that has yet to be fulfilled.

SUMMARY

Veterinary medicine often follows patterns of diagnosis and treatment that have previously been established in human medicine, but it might be that when dealing with brain lesions, specifically tumors, in pet animals, that a different approach is needed. The main reason is cost, as outlined earlier—only a very small proportion of pet owners can afford complicated diagnostic and therapeutic options—and it might perhaps be more appropriate for veterinarians to follow more pragmatic pathways that are more accessible for pet owners.

In such an environment, a prominent role for brain biopsy will continue to be in distinguishing between neoplastic and inflammatory/infectious disease, because these will usually require different therapies. As outlined earlier, it can be difficult to distinguish these 2 processes on images alone. To make the process more accessible to owners, the use of cheap equipment that allows for rapid procedures would be beneficial in terms of more accurate diagnosis and minimal cost. As such, 3D-printed guides may represent the best way forward at present because they are easily created, and the biopsies obtained using such devices have acceptable diagnostic rates.

Brain biopsy will also continue to be an important component of clinical trials in which the efficacy of a specific therapy is investigated, so that effectiveness can be related to the specific lesion category.

DISCLOSURE

The author has nothing to disclose.

REFERENCES

1. Bentley RT. Magnetic resonance imaging diagnosis of brain tumors in dogs. Vet J 2015;205:204–16.

2. May JL, Garcia-Mora J, Edwards M, et al. An Illustrated Scoping Review of the Magnetic Resonance Imaging Characteristics of Canine and Feline Brain Tumors. Animals (Basel) 2024;14:1044.

3. Yan PF, Yan L, Zhang Z, et al. Accuracy of conventional MRI for preoperative diagnosis of intracranial tumors: A retrospective cohort study of 762 cases. Int J Surg 2016;36:109–17.

4. Cervera V, Mai W, Vite CH, et al. Comparative magnetic resonance imaging findings between gliomas and presumed cerebrovascular accidents in dogs. Vet Radiol Ultrasound 2011;52:33–40.

5. Maclellan MJ, Ober CP, Feeney DA, et al. Evaluation of diffusion-weighted magnetic resonance imaging at 3.0 Tesla for differentiation between intracranial neoplastic and noninfectious inflammatory lesions in dogs. J Am Vet Med Assoc 2019;255:71–7.

6. Wanamaker MW, Vernau KM, Taylor SL, et al. Classification of neoplastic and inflammatory brain disease using MRI texture analysis in 119 dogs. Vet Radiol Ultrasound 2021;62:445–54.

7. Stadler KL, Ober CP, Feeney DA, et al. Multivoxel proton magnetic resonance spectroscopy of inflammatory and neoplastic lesions of the canine brain at 3.0 T. Am J Vet Res 2014;75:982–9.

8. Granger N, Smith PM, Jeffery ND. Clinical findings and treatment of non-infectious meningoencephalomyelitis in dogs: a systematic review of 457 published cases from 1962 to 2008. Vet J 2010;184:290–7.

9. Butterfield S, Whittaker D, Tabanez J, et al. Bacterial meningitis secondary to otogenic infection in 10 French bulldogs: A retrospective case series. Vet Rec Open 2023;10:e263.

10. Robson K, Smith PM. Cryptococcal meningoencephalitis in a dog. Vet Rec 2011; 168:538.

11. Jacobson E, Morton JM, Woerde DJ, et al. Clinical features, outcomes, and long-term survival times of cats and dogs with central nervous system cryptococcosis in Australia: 50 cases (2000-2020). J Am Vet Med Assoc 2022;261:246–57.

12. Westworth DR, Dickinson PJ, Vernau W, et al. Choroid plexus tumors in 56 dogs (1985-2007). J Vet Intern Med 2008;22:1157–65.

13. Cluzel C, Aboulmali AA, Dugas S, et al. Diffuse leptomeningeal histiocytic sarcoma in the cerebrospinal fluid of 2 dogs. Vet Clin Pathol 2016;45:184–90.

14. Toyoda I, Vernau W, Sturges BK, et al. Clinicopathological characteristics of histiocytic sarcoma affecting the central nervous system in dogs. J Vet Intern Med 2020;34:828–37.

15. Bailey CS, Higgins RJ. Characteristics of cisternal cerebrospinal fluid associated with primary brain tumors in the dog: a retrospective study. J Am Vet Med Assoc 1986;188:414–6.

16. Dickinson PJ, Sturges BK, Kass PH, et al. Characteristics of cisternal cerebrospinal fluid associated with intracranial meningiomas in dogs: 56 cases (1985-2004). J Am Vet Med Assoc 2006;228:564–7.

17. Louis DN, Perry A, Wesseling P, et al. The 2021 WHO Classification of Tumors of the Central Nervous System: a summary. Neuro Oncol 2021;23:1231–51.

18. Krane GA, Shockley KR, Malarkey DE, et al. Inter-pathologist agreement on diagnosis, classification and grading of canine glioma. Vet Comp Oncol 2022;20: 881–9.

19. Ivan ME, Yarlagadda J, Saxena AP, et al. Brain shift during bur hole-based procedures using interventional MRI. J Neurosurg 2014;121:149–60.

20. Pećina-Šlaus N, Hrašćan R. Glioma stem cells-features for new therapy design. Cancers (Basel) 2024;16:1557.

21. Goel D, Sundaram C, Paul TR, et al. Intraoperative cytology (squash smear) in neurosurgical practice - pitfalls in diagnosis experience based on 3057 samples from a single institution. Cytopathology 2007;18:300–8.

22. Roessler K, Dietrich W, Kitz K. High diagnostic accuracy of cytologic smears of central nervous system tumors. A 15-year experience based on 4,172 patients. Acta Cytol 2002;46:667–74.

23. Vernau KM, Higgins RJ, Bollen AW, et al. Primary canine and feline nervous system tumors: intraoperative diagnosis using the smear technique. Vet Pathol 2001; 38:47–57.

24. Levitin HA, Foss KD, Hague DW, et al. The utility of intraoperative impression smear cytology of intracranial granular cell tumors: Three cases. Vet Clin Pathol 2019;48:282–6.

25. De Lorenzi D, Mandara MT, Tranquillo M, et al. Squash-prep cytology in the diagnosis of canine and feline nervous system lesions: a study of 42 cases. Vet Clin Pathol 2006;35:208–14.

26. Bianconi A, Donada M, Zeppa P, et al. How Reliable Is Fluorescence-Guided Surgery in Low-Grade Gliomas? A Systematic Review Concerning Different Fluorophores. Cancers (Basel) 2023;15:4130.

27. Chang CY, Chen CC. 5-aminolevulinic enhanced brain lesions mimic glioblastoma: A case report and literature review. Medicine (Baltimore) 2024;103:e34518.

28. Policicchio D, Doda A, Sgaramella E, et al. Ultrasound-guided brain surgery: echographic visibility of different pathologies and surgical applications in neurosurgical routine. Acta Neurochir (Wien) 2018;160:1175–85.

29. Adams BS, Marino DJ, Loughin CA, et al. Evaluation of an ultrasound-guided freeze-core biopsy system for canine and feline brain tumors. Front Vet Sci 2024;11:1284097.

30. Somerset HL, Kleinschmidt-DeMasters BK. Approach to the intraoperative consultation for neurosurgical specimens. Adv Anat Pathol 2011;18:446–9.

31. Flegel T, Oevermann A, Oechtering G, et al. Diagnostic yield and adverse effects of MRI-guided free-hand brain biopsies through a mini-burr hole in dogs with encephalitis. J Vet Intern Med 2012;26:969–76.

32. WPI. Available at: https://www.wpiinc.com/var-505269-lab-standard-stereotaxic-instrument.html?gad_source=1&gclid=CjwKCAjw57exBhAsEiwAalxaZiT06AyXv v2EGbB_pAquOuW1kAZ1GFTacg5giJG2pDYwgWZbTkh2kRoCufgQAvD_BwE. Accessed May 1, 2024.

33. Rossmeisl JH, Andriani RT, Cecere TE, et al. Frame-based stereotactic biopsy of canine brain masses: technique and clinical results in 26 cases. Front Vet Sci 2015;2:20.

34. Troxel MT, Vite CH. CT-guided stereotactic brain biopsy using the Kopf stereotactic system. Vet Radiol Ultrasound 2008;49:438–43.

35. Koblik PD, LeCouteur RA, Higgins RJ, et al. CT-guided brain biopsy using a modified Pelorus Mark III stereotactic system: experience with 50 dogs. Vet Radiol Ultrasound 1999;40:434–40.

36. Moissonnier P, Blot S, Devauchelle P, et al. Stereotactic CT-guided brain biopsy in the dog. J Small Anim Pract 2002;43:115–23.

37. Kani Y, Cecere TE, Lahmers K, et al. Diagnostic accuracy of stereotactic brain biopsy for intracranial neoplasia in dogs: Comparison of biopsy, surgical resection, and necropsy specimens. J Vet Intern Med 2019;33:1384–91.

38. Packer RA, Freeman LJ, Miller MA, et al. Evaluation of minimally invasive excisional brain biopsy and intracranial brachytherapy catheter placement in dogs. Am J Vet Res 2011;72:109–21.

39. Flegel T, Podell M, March PA, et al. Use of a disposable real-time CT stereotactic navigator device for minimally invasive dog brain biopsy through a mini-burr hole. AJNR Am J Neuroradiol 2002;23:1160–3.

40. Taylor AR, Cohen ND, Fletcher S, et al. Application and machine accuracy of a new frameless computed tomography-guided stereotactic brain biopsy system in dogs. Vet Radiol Ultrasound 2013;54:332–42.

41. Chen AV, Wininger FA, Frey S, et al. Description and validation of a magnetic resonance imaging-guided stereotactic brain biopsy device in the dog. Vet Radiol Ultrasound 2012;53:150–6.

42. Kaes M, Beynon C, Kiening K, et al. Stereotactic frame-based biopsy of infratentorial lesions via the suboccipital-transcerebellar approach with the Zamorano-Duchovny stereotactic system-a retrospective analysis of 79 consecutive cases. Acta Neurochir (Wien) 2024;166:147.

43. Gutmann S, Tästensen C, Böttcher IC, et al. Clinical use of a new frameless optical neuronavigation system for brain biopsies: 10 cases (2013-2020). J Small Anim Pract 2022;63:468–81.
44. Müller M, Winkler D, Möbius R, et al. A concept for a 3D-printed patient-specific stereotaxy platform for brain biopsy -a canine cadaver study. Res Vet Sci 2019; 124:79–84.
45. Gutmann S, Winkler D, Müller M, et al. Accuracy of a magnetic resonance imaging-based 3D printed stereotactic brain biopsy device in dogs. J Vet Intern Med 2020;34:844–51.
46. Gutmann S, Flegel T, Müller M, et al. Case report: clinical use of a patient-individual magnetic resonance imaging-based stereotactic navigation device for brain biopsies in three dogs. Front Vet Sci 2022;9:876741.
47. Shinn R, Park C, DeBose K, et al. Feasibility and accuracy of 3D printed patient-specific skull contoured brain biopsy guides. Vet Surg 2021;50:933–43.
48. James MD, Bova FJ, Rajon DA, et al. Novel MRI and CT compatible stereotactic brain biopsy system in dogs using patient-specific facemasks. J Small Anim Pract 2017;58:615–21.
49. She C, Sun Z, Zhang Z, et al. Noninvasive targeting system with three-dimensionally printed customized device in stereotactic brain biopsy. World Neurosurg 2024;183:e649–57.
50. Dhawan S, Venteicher AS, Butler WE, et al. Clinical outcomes as a function of the number of samples taken during stereotactic needle biopsies: a meta-analysis. J Neuro Oncol 2021;154:1–11.
51. Shinn RL, Kani Y, Hsu FC, et al. Risk factors for adverse events occurring after recovery from stereotactic brain biopsy in dogs with primary intracranial neoplasia. J Vet Intern Med 2020;34:2021–8.
52. Riche M, Marijon P, Amelot A, et al. Severity, timeline, and management of complications after stereotactic brain biopsy. J Neurosurg 2021;136:867–76.
53. Zhang QJ, Wang WH, Wei XP, et al. Safety and efficacy of frameless stereotactic brain biopsy techniques. Chin Med Sci J 2013;28:113–6.
54. Jozsa F, Gaier C, Ma Y, et al. Safety and efficacy of brain biopsy: Results from a single institution retrospective cohort study. Brain Spine 2023;3:101763.
55. Hu H, Barker A, Harcourt-Brown T, et al. Systematic Review of Brain Tumor Treatment in Dogs. J Vet Intern Med 2015;29:1456–63.
56. Herzig R, Beckmann K, Körner M, et al. A shortened whole brain radiation therapy protocol for meningoencephalitis of unknown origin in dogs. Front Vet Sci 2023;10:1132736.
57. Santos M, Roque R, Rainha Campos A, et al. Impact of brain biopsy on management of nonneoplastic brain disease. Brain Spine 2022;2:100863.
58. Bex A, Mathon B. Advances, technological innovations, and future prospects in stereotactic brain biopsies. Neurosurg Rev 2022;46:5.
59. Pasqualetti F, Rizzo M, Franceschi S, et al. New perspectives in liquid biopsy for glioma patients. Curr Opin Oncol 2022;34:705–12.
60. Marioni-Henry K, Zaho D, Amengual-Batle P, et al. Expression of microRNAs in cerebrospinal fluid of dogs with central nervous system disease. Acta Vet Scand 2018;60:80.
61. Lake BB, Rossmeisl JH, Cecere J, et al. Immunosignature differentiation of non-infectious meningoencephalomyelitis and intracranial neoplasia in dogs. Front Vet Sci 2018;5:97.

Complications in Intracranial Surgery of Companion Animals

Andy Shores, DVM, MS, PhD, DACVIM (Neurology)*,
Michelle L. Mendoza, DVM

KEYWORDS

- Craniectomy/craniotomy • Cerebral edema • Hemorrhage • Aspiration pneumonia
- Seizures

KEY POINTS

- Presurgical and adjunctive therapy plus anesthetic protocol appear to be keys to successful surgery.
- Aspiration pneumonia is among the most common complications.
- Proper preparation in designing the surgical approach, prior experience, and length of surgery are all helpful in avoidance of many complications.
- Serial postoperative monitoring and early return to a nutritional plane are major components in avoiding complications.

INTRODUCTION

The art of intracranial surgery in the canine and feline patients essentially began with the publication of Dr. John Oliver's work in 1968[1] in which he described the surgical approaches to the brain. Most of his approaches are still used today.[2] With the advent and increasing availability of advanced imaging techniques, intracranial surgery has become much more commonplace in the field of veterinary neurosurgery. As our companion animals live longer intracranial mass lesions are becoming more common. Depending on location, size, and type, surgery can be a viable option for owners.

As we continue to expand the utilization of this approach to intracranial maladies in the dog and cat, we are also gaining more experience in avoiding or at least being aware of potential complications. This article addresses many of these and provides some ideas of how they can be avoided when possible.

Department of Clinical Science, College of Veterinary Medicine, Mississippi State Univeristy, 240 Wise Center Drive, Mississippi State, MS 39762, USA
* Corresponding author.
E-mail address: shores@cvm.msstate.edu

Vet Clin Small Anim 55 (2025) 57–66
https://doi.org/10.1016/j.cvsm.2024.07.006   **vetsmall.theclinics.com**
0195-5616/25/© 2024 Elsevier Inc. All rights are reserved, including those for text and data mining, AI training, and similar technologies.

INDICATIONS

The indications for intracranial surgery in companion animals are listed in **Box 1**. Among these are intracranial masses. Meningiomas are the most common brain tumor in canine and feline patients. In one study, intracranial surgery for meningioma resection offers an excellent prognosis for survival to discharge from hospital with a median long-term survival time of 386 days.[3] While meningiomas carry the best prognosis, other tumors can be much more sinister and carry a much poorer prognosis despite treatment, with gliomas often being the most challenging. The overall mortality rate of patients undergoing cranial surgery in one study was 14.5% within 10 days after surgery.[4] Gordon and colleagues[5] reported a mortality rate of 19% for 42 cats undergoing craniotomy for the treatment of cerebral meningioma.

SURGICAL APPROACHES TO THE BRAIN

The 3 most common approaches are the rostrotentorial,[2] transfrontal,[6] and sub-occipital.[7] Additional approaches include transsphenoidal hypophysectomy[8] and the lateral, transzygomatic approach.[9] Illustrations of the 3 most common approaches are shown in **Fig. 1**.

TYPES OF COMPLICATIONS

The more common complications can be characterized as intraoperative and postoperative.

Intraoperative

These complications include brain swelling and hemorrhage and can occur for many reasons including obstruction of outflow, unnecessary trauma to the brain parenchyma caused by surgical manipulation, and poor anesthetic management that diminishes the natural protective effects (autoregulation)—this may include elevated CO_2, over-zealous intravenous (IV) fluid administration, changes in the blood pressure (both increases and decreases outside of a normal range) and some other issues such as metabolic acidosis. Hemorrhage is obviously a result of disruption of vessels within the cranial vault, incomplete or poor surgical planning, and overly aggressive surgical manipulation. Additionally, elevated mean arterial pressure can make hemorrhage more likely and more difficult to control.

Box 1
Indications for intracranial surgery in companion animals

- Head trauma
  - Depressed fractures
  - Penetrating foreign bodies/projectiles
  - Hematoma evacuation
- Intracranial and extracranial masses
  - Neoplasia
  - Abscesses
- Shunt placement and marsupialization
  - Hydrocephalus
  - Quadrigeminal diverticulum
- Chiari-like malformation

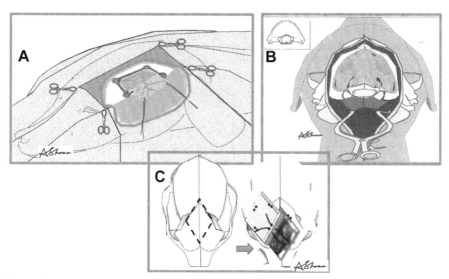

Fig. 1. The 3 most common surgical approaches to the canine brain: (A) rostrotentorial, (B) sub-occipital, and (C) transfrontal. *Images courtesy of* Dr Andy Shores, DVM, MS, PhD, DACVIM (Neurology).

Placement of a ventricular catheter for ventriculoperitoneal shunting or a lateral ventricular fenestration for hydrocephalus can cause a collapse of the cortex. This can occur intraoperatively from a sudden change in pressures or days to weeks postoperatively from over shunting (**Fig. 2**). In addition, hemorrhage underneath the burr hole can create a compressive hematoma.

Postoperative

These complications can be caused by the effects of the surgery (damage to critical areas of the brain, continued brain swelling/edema). An additional concern, and arguably among the most common postoperative complications, is aspiration pneumonia.[10]

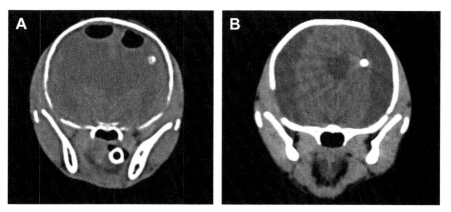

Fig. 2. Bilateral cortical collapse resulting from over-shunting a hydrocephalic patient. Fortunately, the patient did not show severe effects, but many do. (A) Immediate postop and (B) 2 week postop computed tomographic scans showing bilateral cortical collapse.

Continued brain swelling and edema, left unchecked, invariably leads to transtentorial or foramen magnum herniation and most likely death or severe permanent disability. Aspiration pneumonia can be a consequence of pre-existing issues (brachycephalic syndrome, esophagitis, reflux)[10] or issues with prolonged use of postoperative medications designed to manage pain and maintain sedation. Of these, fentanyl is a player, and the combination of fentanyl and benzodiazepams is known to cause respiratory depression and may reduce the swallowing reflex and this creates a condition more conducive to aspiration.[11]

Seizures are also a common postoperative complication and are possibly a pre-existing condition, a new manifestation of the brain disease plus surgery, or less than appropriate anticonvulsant blood levels.

In humans, one reported postoperative complication is ischemic stroke; although the incidence is low without a pre-existing disposition.[12] To our knowledge, this has never been documented in the veterinary literature, but could be a malady that we have never fully evaluated postoperatively in animals. Certain pre-operative conditions that contribute to hypercoagulability certainly can exist in companion animals.

Nutrition plays an important role in the recovery process and the caloric requirements increase substantially after the surgery.[13] An overly sedated patient fed orally also presents another type of opportunity for aspiration.

Depending on the initial indication for the intracranial surgery, one must address the possibility of infection as a potential complication. A bite to the head that penetrates the skull, and abscess that forms in the presence of a systemic infection, from penetration of the cribriform plate, or from any projectile penetrating the skull all are considered an intracranial contamination/infection. Iatrogenic contamination should be highly unlikely in the modern surgical suites, but not impossible. Any transfrontal approach to the brain does expose the cranial vault to the nasal cavities and sinuses and without using some preventative measures is not an uncommon site for postoperative infection.[14]

Postoperative hemorrhage after cranial neurosurgery in humans is a serious complication with substantial morbidity and mortality. This does occur in the veterinary field (**Fig. 3**). Compressive hematomas can be devastating.[15]

An additional complication in the rostrotentorial approach can be herniation of the cerebral cortex through the craniectomy site. This can be transitory as postoperative

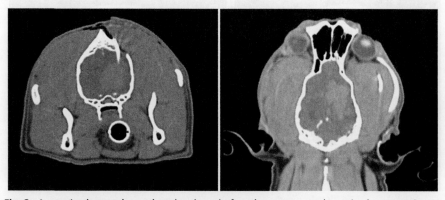

Fig. 3. A massive hemorrhage that developed after the surgery and required reoperation to remove the compressive hematoma and stop the hemorrhage. Shown are axial and dorsal computed tomographic images of the hematoma.

swelling subsides; however, unless there is adequate protection over the site, muscle adhesions to the cerebral cortex can be a long-term complication.

Following a transfrontal approach, sub-cutaneous emphysema, pneumocephalus, and pneumomediastinum are reported complications.[6] While these are usually transient, a tension pneumocephalus or pneumomediastinum can be life-threatening.

PREVENTATIVE MEASURES

Careful pre-surgical planning is a must. This includes a thorough review of the images and collecting a complete pre-surgical minimum data base. It is helpful to have both computed tomographic and MR images for planning. Contrast images are most useful.

The anesthetic protocol is an essential component of this procedure and may be of capital importance in preventing some of the pre-surgical and post-surgical complication. Many anesthetists choose to use an IV anesthetic protocol.[16] Nonetheless, others will use an inhalant for maintenance (isoflurane or sevoflurane)[3] without reported complications. Other iterations include induction with propofol plus lidocaine and combine sevoflurane and either a short-acting opioid or dexmedetomidine for maintenance.[17] Likely, the most important factor is paying attention to the monitoring parameters, especially mean arterial pressure, end-tidal CO_2, and arterial blood gas values. Most of this relates to means to reduce chances of elevated intracranial pressure. Total IV anesthesia carried a better prognosis than inhalant anesthesia according to one study.[4] Compared to inhalant, patients on IV anesthesia with propofol were seen to wake up faster and had decreased intracranial pressure. Volatile inhalant agents are reported by some to interfere with cerebral blood flow regulation, which can lead to an increase in intracranial pressure and decreased cerebral perfusion.[18] Significant increases in intracranial pressure have been reported in animals with intracranial masses and low doses of volatile anesthetic.[19,20] Other authors have reported very good success with inhalants.[3] Another factor to consider is that patients maintained on remifentanil for anesthetic maintenance can develop a postoperative hyperalgesia, and require increased opioids for analgesia and therefore increased sedation postoperatively—this itself can lead to complications and is clearly an indication for a need for multimodal pain medications.[21] Strong consideration to developing anesthetic protocols using dexmedetomidine continuous rate infusions is warranted.

Patients with intracranial lesions typically have increased intracranial pressure which can be a large risk factor perioperatively and postoperatively. Any increase in intracranial pressure can lead to decrease in brain function and ultimately brain herniation.[22] Increased intracranial pressure at the time of induction and intubation can be reduced using IV lidocaine as a component of anesthetic induction. Intracranial pressure hypertension, which was defined as greater than 13 mm Hg 15 minutes after discontinuation of anesthesia, was associated with a poor prognosis in one study.[23] During surgery, intracranial pressure may rise due to surgical manipulation; however, surgical removal of overlying skull and incision of the dura mater can decrease intracranial pressure.[24] Certainly, keeping manipulation to a minimum and avoiding significant hemorrhage are key factors in avoiding issues with intracranial pressure. While most are not able to make direct intracranial pressure measurements, especially postoperatively, preventative measures used include continued use of dexamethasone and (as needed) either mannitol or hypertonic saline injections.

Postoperative sedation protocols vary widely, but the ultimate goal is to have a rapid recovery from anesthesia but to also have a patient that does not become overly excited and potentially hypertensive. Pain should not be a major factor in craniotomy patients; however, the skin incision, muscle dissection, and the periosteum are potential sources of pain. Minimizing the use of postoperative opioids has become somewhat of a theme, and in such combining them with other non-opioids seems logical. Possible combinations can include pre- and post-surgical IV acetaminophen and dexmedetomidine with lower doses of methadone. Ketamine can also be a part of a multimodality postoperative management regime.[17]

From our experience with marsupialization of the ventricle, when the hydrocephalus is extreme, we try to place the opening at 50° to 60° off midline (**Fig. 4**). This is based on some research (unpublished) from computer models that show at these locations, the chances of collapse or the cortex is less likely. With ventricular catheters, over shunting likely occurs because in veterinary neurosurgery, our ability to accurately predict and monitor ventricular pressures in small animals makes the choice of valves mostly guesswork. We often choose *medium flow* valves, but these are not always the appropriate choice. In addition, with these procedures, compressive hematomas can occur as a complication, so meticulous attention to hemostasis is a must.

If the surgeon chooses to make a craniotomy and not a craniectomy during a rostrotentorial approach, we believe this takes away a valuable pressure valve that may help to prevent issues associated with postoperative brain swelling. Instead, these authors prefer to use a polypropylene mesh over the site (**Fig. 5**). This material is light weight and provides a protective cover over the defect but still allows for some postoperative brain swelling. Additionally, it can be placed by simply suturing it to the underside of the temporalis muscle in most cases, although some prefer small titanium screws. Other authors prefer the use of a titanium mesh.[25] The purposes of a mesh are to prevent a very large and soft spot at the craniectomy site and prevent muscle adhesions to the cortical tissue.

Transfrontal craniotomies require careful attention to prevent contamination of the cortex from organisms in the sinus cavity and from the creation of pneumocephalus or subcutaneous emphysema (or rarely pneumomediastinum). In our practice, we use some measures which thus far have been very successful in preventing any of those scenarios. First, after the bone flap is removed and the sinus cavity is exposed,

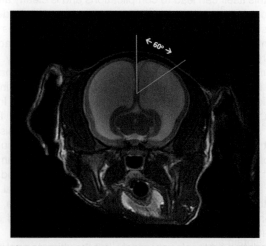

Fig. 4. For patients being treated with a lateral ventricular marsupialization for severe congenital hydrocephalus, we recommend performing the fenestration at a point 50° to 60° from the midline in an effort to avoid cortical collapse.

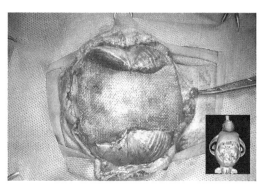

Fig. 5. An example of the use of a polypropylene mesh over a large skull defect in a patient after removal of a skull tumor. The 3 dimensional inset shows the amount of skull removed.

we place a 10% povidone–iodine solution into the sinus cavity and let that sit with the nasal cavity blocked for approximately 10 minutes before suctioning it and flushing the cavity with normal saline. Upon closure, gelatin sponges followed by bone wax are placed into the nasal cavity opening into the sinus and swine-intestinal-submucosa is layered over the exposed frontal cortex. After securing the bone flap, we place bone wax into the gaps between the flap and the rest of the skull to provide somewhat of a seal. In doing these steps, we have not needed to place tubes in the sinuses to prevent air into the calvarium or subcutaneous tissues.

Intraoperative hemorrhage ranges from mild to extreme. In our practice, careful planning of the procedure and the use of intraoperative ultrasound is very helpful in identifying vessels and the occurrence of hemorrhage at the surgery site. Preoperative clotting profiles are standard. Hypertension can also influence the amount of or the development of hemorrhage.

Obviously, seizures are a concern whether they are a preexisting issue or a postoperative event. In our practice, levetiracetam is our go to drug and we ensure it is being administered at an adequate dose and is continued religiously as scheduled, including IV therapy as needed and always at a minimum dose of 30 mg/kg per dose (every 8 hours for regular levetiracetam oral or IV; every 12 hours for extended release). If a patient has not had seizures pre-operatively, we still use levetiracetam prophylactically. If the patient has not had a seizure after 6 months, we try weaning the patient off the medication. In addition, while in the hospital and for the patient at home, intranasal midazolam is available (dose = 0.2 mg/kg) for breakthrough seizures.[20] Our clients are told to use this as often as 4 times in a 2 h span, if needed.

Postoperative vascular events have not been fully evaluated in veterinary neurosurgery. Certainly, there are episodes of postoperative hemorrhage that have been documented, but a brief literature search did not find documented postoperative focal ischemic events. They could be an under diagnosed factor. It is hard to know the causal relationship, but hyperglycemia often develops in people with an ischemic stroke and hyperglycemia following these events seem to correlate with increased risk of death.[26] Additionally, lower potassium levels in people have also been associated with an increased risk of stroke.[27] From this, it seems pertinent to monitor these factors in the postoperative intracranial surgery patient. An additional measure would be to monitor and maintain applicable therapy for patients with renal disease, hyperadrenocorticism, systemic hypertension, and hypothyroidism or hyperthyroidism (in cats) more closely.

Standard protocols for patients with open skull fractures and penetrating wounds is an obvious part of preventing or treating infections—this includes collection of samples for cytology and bacterial culture and sensitivity (aerobic and anaerobic) and instituting appropriate anti-microbial treatment. In certain cases, fungal cultures may also be indicated.[28]

Postoperative nutrition can play a vital role in the recovery of intracranial surgery patients.[13] The likelihood of death for human patients with traumatic brain injury (TBI) who were not fed within 5 days of injury was double that of patients who were fed.[29] In the acute phase of TBI, energy requirements increase to 100%–200% of baseline-predicted resting energy expenditure, and this increase in energy requirement may persist for several weeks to months, depending on the severity of the neurotrauma and level of recovery.[29] When the patient is incapable of or uninterested in eating, IV or tube feeding should be considered as nutrition is an important part of the recovery process.

An important component of postoperative monitoring is serial monitoring and looking for trends in values being measured. Arterial pressures and Pco_2/Po_2/acid–base homeostasis are key. Maintaining an arterial catheter when possible makes obtaining serial blood gas analyses a simpler process.

CONCLUSIONS/DISCUSSION

Intracranial surgery is becoming more common in veterinary neurosurgery, and it seem pertinent to develop sound preanesthetic, anesthetic, and postoperative protocols that are safe and are evidence-based methods that can produce satisfactory outcomes. Currently, the factors we feel are some of the keys to avoiding intraoperative complications include experience of the surgeon and the anesthetist, a carefully planned procedure that limits excessive manipulation, and completing the procedure in a timely manner. Concerning the care of the intracranial surgery patient postoperatively, there are several important factors. Following anesthesia, weaning off ventilatory support as soon as is practical is important as is maintaining the airway. Arterial pressures should be closely monitored, and fluid/electrolyte balances maintained. Blood glucose should also be serially monitored. Providing effective, but balanced analgesia remains a key component of postoperative care. Medications and practices to help control nausea and vomiting are very important. Commencement of early feeding (return to a strong nutritional plane) is a part of that formula.[15] The preoperative and postoperative use of maropitant seems pertinent; however, this does not prevent the overly sedated patients from aspirating some oral secretions. Much can be said for reducing gastric acidity and establishing oral intake as early as possible.

For pain and sedation protocols, the authors strongly recommend a multi-modality approach that limits the amount of opioids. This can include IV acetaminophen (preoperatively and postoperatively), dexmedetomidine, and ketamine in addition to a low dose of an opioid such as methadone.

Careful and continuous postoperative monitoring is essential to head off impending complications. Return to ambulation, when possible, helps in many ways.

CLINICS CARE POINTS

- Sound preanesthetic, anesthetic, and postopertaive protocols are key elements in avoiding complications.

- Careful monitoring will often provide valuable information on the well-being of the patient and signal when additional interventional procedures may be necessary.

DISCLOSURE

The authors have nothing to disclose.

REFERENCES

1. Oliver JE. Surgical approached to the canine brain. Am J Vet Res 1968;29: 353–78.
2. Shores A. Lateral (rostrotentorial) craniotomy/craniectomy. In: Shores A, Brisson B, editors. Current techniques in canine and feline neurosurgery. Hoboken, NJ: John Wiley and Sons; 2017. p. 109–14.
3. Forward AK, Volk HA, Cherubini GB, et al. Clinical presentation, diagnostic findings and outcome of dogs undergoing surgical resection for intracranial meningioma: 101 dogs. BMC Vet Res 2022;18:88.
4. Morton BA, Selmic LE, Vitale S, et al. Indications, complications, and mortality rate following craniotomy or craniectomy in dogs and cats: 165 cases (1995–2016). Journal of the American Veterinary Medical Association 2022;260(9): 1048–56.
5. Gordon LE, Thacher C, Matthiesen DT, et al. Results of craniotomy for the treatment of cerebral meningioma in 42 cats. Vet Surg 1994;23(2):94–100.
6. Uriarte A, Cappello R. Transfrontal craniotomy. In: Shores A, Brisson B, editors. Current techniques in canine and feline neurosurgery. Hoboken, NJ: John Wiley and Sons; 2017. p. 99–107.
7. Akin EY, Shores A. Suboccipital craniectomy/foramen magnum decompression. In: Shores A, Brisson B, editors. Current techniques in canine and feline neurosurgery. Hoboken, NJ: John Wiley and Sons; 2017. p. 115–20.
8. Owen T, Chen-Allen A, Martin L. Surgical management of sellar masses. In: Shores A, Brisson B, editors. Advanced techniques in canine and feline neurosurgery. Hoboken, NJ: John Wiley and Sons; 2023. p. 190–210.
9. Young M, Chen S. Transzygomatic approach to ventrolateral craniotomy/craniectomy. In: Shores A, Brisson B, editors. Advanced techniques in canine and feline neurosurgery. Hoboken, NJ: John Wiley and Sons; 2023. p. 262–6.
10. Fransson BA, Bagley RS, Gay JM, et al. Pneumonia after intracranial surgery in dogs. Vet Surg 2001 Sep-Oct;30(5):432–9. PMID: 11555818.
11. Boon M, van Dorp E, Broens S, et al. Combining opioids and benzodiazepines: effects on mortality and severe adverse respiratory events. Ann Palliat Med 2020;9(2):542–57. Epub 2020 Feb 6. PMID: 32036672.
12. Khan NR, Moore K, Basma J, et al. Ischemic stroke following elective craniotomy in children. J Neurosurg Pediatr 2018;23(3):355–62. PMID: 30579265.
13. Kurtz P, Rocha Eduardo EM. Nutrition Therapy, Glucose Control, and Brain Metabolism in Traumatic Brain Injury: A Multimodal Monitoring Approach. Front Neurosci 2020;14. Available at: https://www.frontiersin.org/journals/neuroscience/articles/10.3389/fnins.2020.00190DOI=10.3389/fnins.2020.00190.
14. Bentley RT. Surgical management of intracranial meningiomas. In: Shores A, Brisson B, editors. Advanced techniques in canine and feline neurosurgery. Hoboken, NJ: John Wiley and Sons; 2023. p. 223–40.

15. Errico Michael, Luoma Astrl MV. Postoperative care of neurosurgical patients: general principles. Anaesth Intensive Care Med 2023;24(Issue 5):282–90.
16. Natalini CC. Practice and principles of neuroanesthesia for imaging and neuro-surgery. In: Shores A, Brisson B, editors. Advanced techniques in canine and fe-line neurosurgery. Hoboken, NJ: John Wiley and Sons; 2023. p. 39–44.
17. Marquez-Grados F, Vettorato E, Corletto F. Sevoflurane with opioid or dexmede-tomidine infusions in dogs undergoing intracranial surgery: a retrospective obser-vational study. J Vet Sci 2020;21(1):e8. https://doi.org/10.4142/jvs.2020.21.e8. PMID: 31940687; PMCID: PMC7000903.
18. Raisis AL, Leece EA, Platt SR, et al. Evaluation of an anaesthetic technique used in dogs undergoing craniectomy for tumour resection. Vet Anaesth Analg 2007; 34(3):171–80.
19. De Decker S, Davies E, Benigni L, et al. Surgical treatment of intracranial epider-moid cyst in a dog: intracranial epidermoid cyst. Vet Surg 2012;41(6):766–77.
20. Charalambous M, Volk HA, Tipold A, et al. Comparison of intranasal versus intra-venous midazolam for management of status epilepticus in dogs: A multi-center randomized parallel group clinical study. J Vet Intern Med 2019;33(6):2709–17. Epub 2019 Oct 3. PMID: 31580527; PMCID: PMC6872604.
21. Yu EH, Tran DH, Lam SW, et al. Remifentanil tolerance and hyperalgesia: short-term gain, long-term pain? Anaesthesia 2016;71(11):1347–62. PMID: 27734470.
22. Kornegay JN, Oliver JE Jr, Gorgacz EJ. Clinicopathologic features of brain herni-ation in animals. J Am Vet Med Assoc 1983;182:1111–6.
23. Seki S, Teshima K, Ito D, et al. Impact of intracranial hypertension on the short-term prognosis in dogs undergoing brain tumor surgery. J Vet Med Sci 2019; 81(8):1205–10. Epub 2019 Apr 12. PMID: 30982789; PMCID: PMC6715920.
24. Bagley RS, Harrington ML, Pluhar GE, et al. Effect of craniectomy/durotomy alone and in combination with hyperventilation, diuretics, and corticosteroids on intra-cranial pressure in clinically normal dogs. Am J Vet Res 1996;57:116–9.
25. Bordelon JT, Rochat MC. Use of a titanium mesh for cranioplasty following radical rostrotentorial craniectomy to remove an ossifying fibroma in a dog. J Am Vet Med Assoc 2007;231(11):1692–5.
26. Kagansky N, Levy S, Knobler H. The Role of Hyperglycemia in Acute Stroke. Arch Neurol 2001;58(8):1209–12.
27. Anxin W, Shuang C, Xue T, et al. Lower Serum Potassium Levels at Admission are Associated with the Risk of Recurrent Stroke in Patients with Acute Ischemic Stroke or Transient Ischemic Attack. Cerebrovasc Dis 2022;51(3):304–12.
28. Pilkington EJ, De Decker S, Mojarradi A, et al. Sinonasal mycosis following trans-frontal craniotomy in three dogs. J Am Vet Med Assoc 2022;260(6):643–9. PMID: 34986118.
29. McClave SA, Martindale RG, Vanek VW, et al. Guidelines for the provision and assessment of nutrition support therapy in the adult critically ill patient: Society of Critical Care Medicine (SCCM) and American Society for Parenteral and Enteral Nutrition (ASPEN). J Parenter Enteral Nutr 2009;33(3):277–316.

Radiation Therapy for Brain Tumors in Dogs and Cats

Tracy L. Gieger, DVM

KEYWORDS

- Radiotherapy • Stereotactic radiosurgery • Brain tumors • Radiobiology
- Central nervous system tumors

KEY POINTS

- Use of external beam radiation therapy (RT) is indicated for non-resectable or incompletely excised brain tumors in dogs and cats.
- Although most patients tolerate RT and improve clinically after treatment, some patients can experience side effects that can be difficult to distinguish from disease progression.
- Anti-seizure therapy and/or steroids may need to be continued indefinitely after the diagnosis of a brain tumor and treatment with RT due to the possibility of ongoing neurologic abnormalities.

INTRODUCTION

External beam radiation therapy (RT) has become the standard of care as a sole treatment for non-resectable or post-operatively for brain tumors in veterinary patients due to its relatively low side effect profile and increasing availability.[1–11] RT delivers ionizing radiation to tumors or regions of the body (such as whole-brain irradiation) to attempt to improve local disease control or delay or prevent post-operative tumor recurrence. At a cellular level, mechanisms of action of ionizing radiation include creating DNA damage (causing cells with unrepaired DNA double strand breaks to lose reproductive capacity and undergo a so-called mitotic death) and inducing interphase death (apoptosis, as is the case with lymphocytes).[3] Clinically, RT prescriptions are delivered in Gray (Gy) and consist of a total dose of RT divided into fractional doses, or "fractions."

It should be noted that most brain tumors in dogs and cats are diagnosed and subsequently treated with RT based on imaging characteristics rather than a tissue diagnosis due to the costs and risks associated with brain biopsies. In a study documenting MRI characteristics versus necropsy findings in dogs with brain tumors, the MRI diagnosis was correct in 70% of patients with primary brain tumors (those arising from the central nervous system [CNS]) and in 93% of secondary brain tumors (including metastasis to the brain from distant sites and tumors of nearby structures

Department of Clinical Sciences, College of Veterinary Medicine, North Carolina State University, 1060 William Moore Drive, Raleigh, NC 27607, USA
E-mail address: tlgieger@ncsu.edu

https://doi.org/10.1016/j.cvsm.2024.07.007
0195-5616/25/© 2024 Elsevier Inc. All rights reserved, including those for text and data mining, AI training, and similar technologies.
vetsmall.theclinics.com

that invade into the calvarium).[12] In a study of cats, the correlation between MRI findings and histopathology was correct 82% of the time.[13]

INDICATIONS FOR RADIATION THERAPY IN DOGS AND CATS WITH BRAIN TUMORS

RT is indicated for the treatment of primary brain tumors (see later for specific tumor types) that are non-resectable (with the goal of trying to prevent tumor progression; tumors may or may not shrink), or post-operatively (with the goal of trying to prevent tumor recurrence).[2–11,14] Secondary brain tumors (most reported to be hemangiosarcoma, and carcinomas), inflammatory diseases (meningoencephalitis of unknown origin [MUO]), and multifocal cancers such as CNS lymphoma and histiocytic sarcoma can also be treated with RT; in these cases, RT is often used concurrently with systemic chemotherapy (for suspected or confirmed multifocal intracranial neoplasia) or immunomodulating drugs (for MUO).[15–18]

PATIENT EVALUATION AND SYSTEMIC STAGING PRIOR TO RADIATION THERAPY

Prior to considering a course of RT, a thorough discussion with the pet owner regarding their goals, budget (for both money and time), possible side effects, and likely outcomes of treatment should be completed by the radiation oncology (RO) clinical team. This client communication is critical since most patients require lifelong continued at-home monitoring, and neurologic improvement (including seizure control) may be gradual over weeks or months after RT (or may not occur at all).[19] Further, late side effects from RT can cause clinical signs that can look like progressive disease.[20,21]

Complete baseline physical and neurologic examinations and a minimum database (ie, complete blood count [CBC], chemistry panel, urinalysis) should be completed to assess for comorbidities that may preclude anesthesia or require further investigation. Additionally, since unrelated primary tumors (different histopathology than the brain tumor, located anywhere in the body) have been reported to occur in >20% of dogs with primary brain tumors, imaging of the abdomen and thorax is recommended prior to finalizing a treatment plan.[22]

RADIATION THERAPY

Colloquially, "definitive-intent RT" is used to describe a course of RT that is anticipated to help control the tumor and associated clinical signs for 1 year or longer, and "palliative-intent RT" (pRT) is used to describe a course of RT that is primarily intended to provide pain control and improvement of clinical signs for a shorter period, without necessarily improving tumor control. In many cases, the distinction between these classifications is difficult in patients with large tumors and persistent or severe neurologic abnormalities. Consultation with a radiation oncologist is recommended to discuss specific recommended treatment options for a specific patient's tumor and overall scenario.

Definitive-intent RT options are most often recommended in patients with brain tumors since they provide the best chance for long-term tumor control. This may be delivered as traditional fractionated RT (FRT; 10–20 daily fractions delivering a total dose of RT ranging from 40 to 50 Gy, Monday–Friday) or stereotactic RT (SRT; 1–5 daily fractions delivering a total dose of RT ranging from 15 to 35 Gy).[4,5,8,9,23–34] Stereotactic RT has the advantage of delivering an intensive course of RT in fewer anesthetic episodes, which is appealing to clinicians and pet owners. The primary downsides of SRT are the need for a well-defined tumor on imaging (since the falloff of dose is only a few mm away from the target and a geographic miss of the tumor could occur if the tumor falls outside of the targeted treatment volume) and a possible increased incidence of early delayed or late effects of RT (see later for a discussion about side effects).[2,3,11] Fractionated RT may be recommended for large, poorly defined tumors or postoperatively if tumors are incompletely excised.[14] Additionally, for patients with pituitary tumors, FRT may be recommended over SRT by some RO team members since the longest published survival times exist for that modality (see pituitary tumors article).

Occasionally, palliative-intent RT protocols may be utilized (typically 4–5 daily or 4–5 once-weekly fractions) delivering a modest total dose of RT (usually 10–24 Gy total dose), but this is anecdotally less common in brain tumor irradiation than with other tumor types.[6] This modality is most often selected for patients with large tumors, severe clinical signs, and/or comorbid conditions.

Whole brain or whole CNS irradiation may be indicated in some cases such as inflammatory diseases, multifocal cancers such as CNS lymphoma, or multifocal metastatic primary brain tumors such as choroid plexus carcinomas.[15–18]

General anesthesia is required for patients undergoing RT to immobilize them for the duration of positioning, pre-treatment image verification ("image-guided radiotherapy"), and treatment (typically 10–30 minutes total for each treatment, or "fraction"). When indicated and if possible, patients should be initially stabilized with glucocorticoids and/or antiseizure medications prior to anesthesia for imaging and RT.

RADIATION TREATMENT PLANNING FOR BRAIN TUMORS

Radiation treatment plans for brain tumors are almost always computer-based RT plans that are created by co-registering computed tomography (CT) scans and MRIs in the radiation treatment planning system (TPS). The goal of treatment planning is to ensure inclusion of gross tumor (GTV, or gross tumor volume), and any suspected adjacent microscopic disease or surgically disrupted areas (CTV, or clinical target volume). When FRT is the planned treatment modality, dosing is based on normal tissue tolerance of the brain adjacent to the GTV and CTV; practically, this means that treatment fields are usually drawn to encompass the GTV and CTV plus 0.3 to 10 mm of surrounding normal tissue to account for interfraction and intrafraction motion (PTV

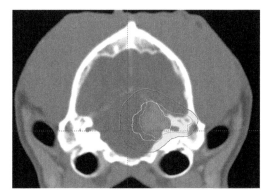

Fig. 1. Transverse computed tomography (CT) scan demonstrating target contours for pre-operative gross tumor volume (GTV), contoured in blue; post-operative GTV, contoured in pink; and the resultant planning target volume (PTV), outlined in purple, which encompasses both structures with a 3 to 5 mm margin that allows for intra-fraction and inter-fraction patient motion. This patient would be treated with a fractionated radiation therapy protocol, consisting of 10-20 daily treatments (total dose 40-50 Gy), Monday-Friday.

or planning target volume) (**Fig. 1**). With SRT, large doses of radiation are carefully sculpted to match the shape of the GTV and then delivered with extreme accuracy (stereotaxis), and with a steep radiation dose gradient that escalates dose in the target, while minimizing dose in adjacent healthy tissues.[35] With SRT, the PTV is typically 0 to 2 mm (**Fig. 2**).[2,3]

In most cases, for brain tumors, the use of intensity-modulated radiation therapy (IMRT, which allows dose intensity to vary across a treatment field) is utilized over simpler treatment modalities such as 3-dimensional conformal radiation therapy (3D CRT, in which all tissues in the field receive the same RT dose) due to the number of critical normal tissues (OAR, or organs-at-risk) adjacent to the brain. Immediately prior to delivery of an RT plan, the patient is imaged using either planar (orthogonal portal images or kilovoltage radiographs obtained from an on-board imaging device [OBI]) or volumetric (ie, cone-beam CT scan [CBCT]) imaging to verify their position relative to the treatment plan, and they are shifted manually or with the use of a robotic couchtop if needed to achieve accurate positioning.[2,36]

CLINICAL FOLLOW-UP AND MONITORING AFTER RADIATION THERAPY

In most patients, lifelong follow-up is required since brain tumors are rarely curable, and clinical signs often recur even after a long period of improvement. The frequency of follow-up visits depends on the patient's diagnosis, comorbidities, specific treatment, and initial response to treatment. At minimum, recheck physical and neurologic examinations are recommended at 3-month to 4-month intervals to monitor clinical signs and to assess quality of life. Repeat imaging of brain tumors after treatment can be considered at 3-month to 6-month intervals to help monitor for tumor recurrence and/or progression, though costs of imaging and risks associated with general anesthesia often preclude pet owners from pursuing this plan. Re-irradiation of brain tumors if the tumor initially responds then progresses is uncommon (but can be considered in some cases) due to the concern of side effects to the normal brain adjacent to the tumor.

For patients with seizures as part of their presenting clinical signs leading to a diagnosis of brain tumors, continued therapy with antiseizure medications should be continued during and after RT (anecdotally, for at least 1 year after the last seizure).

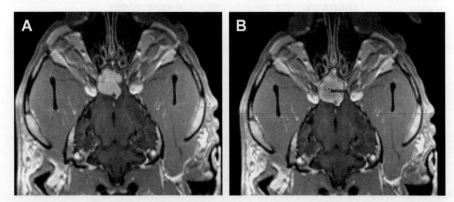

Fig. 2. MRI of a dog with an olfactory menigioma. (*A*) Dorsal plane MRI showing the GTV contoured in red. (*B*) Dorsal plane MRI with the GTV contoured in red and a dose in colorwash showing the dose at 20 Gy. This patient was treated with a 10 Gy × 2 stereotactic radiation therapy protocol, and a simultaneous integrated boost to 25 to 26 Gy was prescribed to the center of the tumor (central red/orange region); the PTV was 0 mm.

Although RT is not a treatment for seizures, RT will hopefully result in slowing of tumor progression and edema surrounding a tumor. One publication compared medical management alone versus the addition of RT in dogs with seizures caused by brain tumors, and the dogs treated with RT had increased time relief from seizures (mean, 24 months with RT vs 2 months without) and survival times (mean, 35 months with RT vs 6 months without).[19]

POTENTIAL ADVERSE EFFECTS ASSOCIATED WITH RADIATION THERAPY

RT-associated side effects are difficult to definitively diagnose due to their intracranial nature; externally visible side effects such as hair loss/haircoat changes and skin hyperpigmentation are occasionally seen but are rarely clinically significant. Side effects associated with RT can be categorized as follows:[2,3,20,21]

- Peracute (within 48 hours of treatment; rare): periprocedural seizures, mentation changes, non-recovery from anesthesia
- Acute (1–6 weeks after RT; occasional): owner-reported somnolence that often responds to an increase in steroid dose
- Early delayed (1–6 months after RT): seizures, neurologic decline that typically responds to treatment with steroids, but can rarely be fatal. This type of adverse effect may be more common with SRT as compared to FRT, since 2 publications report that approximately one-third of dogs receiving SRT for intracranial meningioma experience neurologic decline in the first 6 months after treatment.[20,21]
- Late side effects (>6 months-years after RT; rare): seizures, mentation changes, secondary tumor formation

It is also important to note that both early-delayed and late RT-associated side effects can result in similar clinical signs as tumor progression; therefore, imaging should be used to attempt to differentiate between the 2. In some cases, the presence of edema and white matter changes that are seen after RT may be impossible to differentiate from tumor progression.

GENERAL PROGNOSIS OF DOGS AND CATS WITH BRAIN TUMORS TREATED WITH RADIATION THERAPY

Most dogs and cats with brain tumors will ultimately die or are euthanized due to progression of neurologic disease. In dogs treated with medical management alone (ie, anti-epileptic therapy ± glucocorticoids and pain medication), published survival times range from <1 to 6 months. Dogs with infratentorial tumors and those with severe neurologic signs had poorer outcomes.[37,38] In a study of dogs with various primary brain tumors and neurologic disease treated with RT in addition to medical management, the disease-specific survival time was 699 days, and neither tumor size nor location affected outcome.[4] In a study of cats with various primary brain tumors (primarily suspected meningiomas and pituitary tumors) treated with RT alone, the overall median survival time (MST) was 515 days, with 56% of cats being free of neurologic disease progression at 1 year after treatment.[5] Based on these publications, it is generally accepted that RT will prolong and potentially improve the quality of life for most patients with brain tumors as compared to medical management alone.

MENINGIOMAS IN DOGS

Since meningiomas are extra-axial tumors located between the skull and brain parenchyma, they are the brain tumor type that is most amenable to surgical debulking or resection; therefore, they are occasionally treated with RT in a post-operative setting.[10,14] In a study of dogs treated with surgery followed by FRT, the MST was 16.5 months, as compared to 7 months with surgery alone.[14] It is unclear whether surgery improves survival over FRT alone, since in a different publication, survival times did not differ between groups (FRT alone vs surgery then FRT).[32] Indications for surgery are best assessed by a neurosurgeon, but may include severe neurologic abnormalities or refractory seizures, where craniotomy and tumor debulking may improve clinical signs.

If surgery is not recommended or is declined, RT alone can be a consideration and is widely reported on in the literature. Most publications describe FRT, with MST ranging from 19 to 25 months.[4,8,31,32,34] Stereotactic RT has also been utilized (**Table 1**; see **Fig. 2**).[9,21,33] In a study of dogs with presumed meningiomas treated with SRT, the overall MST was 519 days, with 57% of dogs experiencing a clinical benefit (ie, improvement of clinical signs) after treatment. In that study, 64% of dogs were alive 1 year after RT and 24% were alive 2 years after RT. Dogs with infratentorial tumors had a shorter survival time.[20]

MENINGIOMAS IN CATS

Since meningiomas in cats occur primarily in supratentorial locations, surgery is often performed as the primary treatment. In a study of cats treated with surgery alone, a perioperative mortality rate of 13% was documented, and the overall MST of cats treated in this manner was 37 months.[41] Post-operative recurrence is possible, though objective information on the incidence of and timeframe to recurrence is lacking, since meningiomas are typically slow-growing and may not be reimaged after surgery unless or until clinical signs recur. Cats can be treated with FRT post-operatively or with FRT or SRT if surgery is not possible, but publications regarding long-term outcomes are lacking; anecdotally, outcomes are thought to be like that of dogs.

GLIOMAS IN DOGS

In many cases, the presence of edema surrounding a presumed glioma can provide a challenge for the RO team during treatment planning (distinguishing edema from tumor); therefore, in some cases, a recheck MRI after a 2 to 3-week course of steroids may be warranted to improve target delineation prior to RT. Gliomas in dogs may be treated with RT alone or surgery followed by RT, though publications describing the latter are lacking. In contrast to historical publications documenting poorer outcomes in dogs with gliomas, numerous recent publications describing FRT or SRT have documented MST of 1 to 2 years (see **Table 1**).[24–26,39] In a study, the addition of chemotherapy improved survival time (MST >658 days vs 230 days without chemotherapy); in addition, some dogs were treated with multiple courses of SRT, further prolonging their survival.[39] In a study of dogs treated with FRT, dogs whose tumors contacted the subventricular zone had a higher rate of disease progression and a shorter survival time.[25]

Gliomas are uncommon in cats, and a single publication documented treatment of a cat with FRT (survival time was 575 days after FRT).[5,42,43]

CHOROID PLEXUS TUMORS IN DOGS (RARE IN CATS)

Intraventricular tumors such as ependymomas and choroid plexus tumors (classified as papilloma, atypical papilloma, or carcinoma) are relatively uncommon in dogs and are rare in cats.[22,23,43,44] They have the potential to seed the ventricular system via

Table 1
Summary of recent publications regarding stereotactic radiation therapy for intracranial tumors in dogs

Reference	Tumor Type	# Dogs	Radiation Prescription(s)	Overall Survival Time	Toxicity	Comments
Hansen et al,[23] 2023	Intraventricular tumors	11	8 Gy × 3 = 24 Gy 15 Gy × 1 = 15 Gy	Median 151 d (95% CI 33–1593)	None reported; 2/11 dogs were euthanized within 6 wk of SRT	6/11 had biopsy confirmation of choroid plexus papilloma or carcinoma or ependymoma
Trageser et al,[24] 2023	Glioma	23	16 or 18 Gy × 1 = 16–18 Gy 8 Gy × 3 = 24 Gy 6.75 × 4 = 27 Gy	Median 349 d (95% CI 162–584) Median disease-specific survival time 413 d (95% CI 217–717)	3/23 dogs living >180 d after SRT had suspected late side effects	21/23 dogs had improvement in clinical signs after SRT; 13/23 dogs were brachycephalic
Moirano et al,[39] 2020	Glioma	21	8–9.5 × 3 = 24–27 Gy	Median 636 d	3/21 had presumed acute toxicity that responded to steroids	7/21 had additional courses of SRT, and median survival time of those dogs was >866 d; dogs that had chemotherapy had longer survival times
Swift et al,[28] 2017	Trigeminal nerve sheath tumor	27 dogs (15 treated with SRT)	8 Gy × 3 = 24 Gy 10 Gy × 3 = 30 Gy	Median 441 d (95% CI 260–518) for dogs treated with SRT	Some dogs developed facial pain after treatment	Due to overlap in the 95% CI between treated and untreated dogs, unknown benefit of SRT as compared to no treatment; clinical signs such as facial pain and ocular deficits did not resolve after treatment in most dogs

(continued on next page)

Table 1
(continued)

Reference	Tumor Type	# Dogs	Radiation Prescription(s)	Overall Survival Time	Toxicity	Comments
Dolera et al,[27] 2018	Trigeminal nerve sheath tumor	7	7.4 Gy × 5 = 37 Gy	Median 952 d (95% CI, 543–1361d)	None reported	MRI after treatment in all dogs; 1 CR, 4 PR, 2 SD; 4/7 dogs had extracranial extension of the tumor; clinical signs did not resolve in most dogs
Hansen et al,[29] 2016	Trigeminal nerve sheath tumor	8	8 Gy × 3 = 24 Gy	Median 324 d (95% CI: 99–975)	None reported. 6/8 dogs were euthanized due to seizures and progressive neurologic signs, and the remaining 2 dogs experienced accident-related death	Median disease-specific survival time: 745 d
Dolera et al,[20] 2018	Glioma	42	4.2 Gy × 10 = 42 Gy 5.3 Gy × 7 = 37 Gy 6.6 Gy × 5 = 33 Gy 7 Gy × 5 = 35 Gy	RT alone: 50% alive at 1 y, 41% at 2 y RT + TMZ: 65% alive at 1 y, 40% at 2 y	Minimal	Radiation dose was scaled based on tumor grade and volume 22 dogs RT alone; 20 RT + TMZ; no difference in outcomes; RT dose based on size of tumor relative to normal brain
Griffin et al,[21] 2016	Meningioma	30	8 Gy × 3 = 24 Gy	Median 561 d (95% CI 423–875d), 60.8% 1 y survival, 33.2% 2 y	37% worsened neurologically 3–16 wk after SRT, 13% died of neurologic progression within 6 mo	Volume of normal brain treated predicted death

Study	Tumor	Number	Dose	Survival	Toxicity	Notes
Kelsey et al,[20] 2018	Meningioma	32	16 Gy × 1 = 16 Gy	Median 519 d (95% CI 330–708d), 64% 1 y survival, 24% 2 y	31% worsened neurologically within 6 mo after SRT; 10% died of neurologic progression	Infratentorial tumors and higher gradient index predicted shorter survival time
Dolera et al,[33] 2018	Meningioma	39 (33 with encephalic meningioma, 6 spinal meningioma)	6.6 Gy × 5 = 33 Gy	2-y overall survival: 74.3%	1 dog had mild neurotoxicity	2-y disease-specific survival: 97.4% 49% of dogs had a partial or complete response at 2 y, when considering both objective follow-up imaging data and clinical status in response evaluation.

Abbreviations: CR, complete response, disappearance of all target lesions[40]. d, days; Gy, Gray; MRI, magnetic resonance imaging; PR, partial response–30% or greater decrease in the sum diameters of target lesions[40]; RT, radiation therapy; SD, stable disease–less than 30% reduction or up to 20% increase in the sum diameters of target lesions[40]; SRT, stereotactic radiation therapy; TMZ, temozolomide.

normal flow of cerebrospinal fluid (CSF), forming "drop metastases" at sites distant from the main mass. Ideally, for patients with suspected choroid plexus tumors, baseline staging tests including both CSF analysis and MRI of the entire brain and spine are recommended. If the disease is confined to the brain at the time of diagnosis, FRT or SRT may be considered. If multifocal CNS lesions are present, entire craniospinal irradiation and/or chemotherapy could be considered. There is no standard RT approach, and the literature is scant on outcomes with RT.[23] In one study of 11 dogs treated with SRT (see **Table 1**), the MST was 515 days, and the majority of dogs had a clinical benefit from treatment; however, 4/11 dogs were euthanized within 7 weeks of treatment. Two dogs with biopsy-confirmed choroid plexus carcinomas had survival times of 24 and 133 days.

TRIGEMINAL NERVE SHEATH TUMORS IN DOGS (RARE IN CATS)

Trigeminal nerve sheath tumors are often diagnosed during a workup for masseter muscle atrophy (**Fig. 3**) and can cause a mass effect at the brainstem with possible extension along all 3 peripheral branches of the nerve (maxillary, mandibular, ophthalmic).[45] Radiation is primarily used as a sole treatment for this disease due to its location. Three studies reported on use of SRT in a total of 30 dogs with TNST.[27–29] The median survival times ranged from 441 to 952 days, and anecdotally, similar outcomes are observed with FRT. In a study, 4/5 dogs with clinical signs related to intracranial disease improved, but peripheral neuropathies (facial pain, muscle atrophy) did not improve in most cases and 6/15 dogs had persistent poor ocular health after treatment.[28] It is therefore critical to educate pet owners about the goals of this treatment—that is, an attempt to slow down disease progression for both the intracranial and extracranial components of the disease, without a robust expectation that the externally visible clinical signs will improve.

MULTILOBULAR TUMOR OF BONE AND OTHER CALVARIAL TUMORS

Neoplasms of the skull such as multilobular tumor of bone (MLO) and osteosarcoma can cause compression of the brain (**Fig. 4**) and result in neurologic dysfunction. Radiation therapy often plays a role in multimodal therapy due to tumor location and inability to perform complete surgical excision (see **Fig. 4**). In a recent series of 8

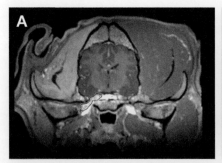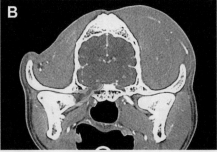

Fig. 3. MRI of the brain of a dog with a trigeminal nerve sheath tumor. (*A*) Transverse T1 post contrast image. The extra-cranial and intra-cranial aspects are contoured in red (gross tumor volume, GTV). (*B*)Transverse T1 post contrast image. Both extra-cranial and intracranial aspects are contoured in red (gross tumor volume, GTV) and a dose in colorwash is showing the dose at 30 Gy. This patient was treated with a 10 Gy × 3 stereotactic radiation therapy protocol.

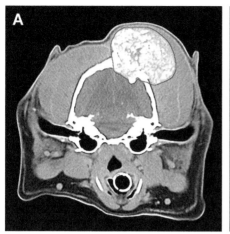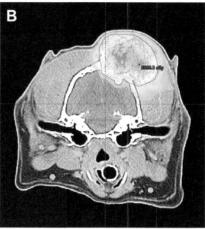

Fig. 4. Transverse computed tomography showing a multilobular tumor of bone. (*A*) The GTV is contoured in red. (*B*) The GTV is contoured in red and dose in colorwash is showing the dose ranging from 20 Gy adjacent to the normal brain (*green*) to 30 Gy (yellow), up to a nearly 40 Gy simultaneous integrated boost at the center of the tumor (*red*). This patient was treated with a 10 Gy × 3 stereotactic radiation therapy protocol.

dogs treated with SRT as the sole treatment, the overall median survival time was 329 days, and 4/5 dogs that were reimaged with CT scans had a 26% to 87% reduction in tumor volume.[30] It is important to perform both CT and MRI in such cases to assess the bony extent (CT scan) and intracranial soft tissue extent (MRI) of these masses for RT planning purposes.[30] When surgical margins are narrow and/or incomplete, adjunctive FRT can be used to reduce risk of local recurrence.[46,47] In a case series of 3 dogs treated with surgical excision of the tumor followed by FRT (2.5 Gy × 22 fractions), survival times ranged from 358 to 677 days.[46]

NON-NEOPLASTIC INFLAMMATORY DISEASE AND MULTIFOCAL CENTRAL NERVOUS SYSTEM NEOPLASIA

Dogs with MUO may benefit from the use of RT in addition to medical management.[17,18] In a pilot study of 6 dogs which received a total dose of 30 Gy in 10 fractions (whole brain), plus corticosteroids at immunosuppressive doses, all patients showed clinical improvement, with 5/6 surviving for >12 months after RT.[17] Another study from the same group reported on outcomes of 10 dogs treated with a shorter protocol (4 Gy × 5); all of those dogs improved clinically with no known RT side effects, and the MST was 723 days (CI 436–1011 days).[18] Whole brain irradiation using similar doses may also be considered in patients with multifocal neoplastic brain disease (such as lymphoma, histiocytic sarcoma), although a paucity of information exists in the literature.[15,16,43]

DISCLOSURE

Dr T.L. Gieger does not have relevant commercial or financial conflicts of interest, or funding sources which are relevant to this article.

REFERENCES

1. Dunfield EM, Turek MM, Buhr KA, et al. A survey of stereotactic radiation therapy in veterinary medicine. Vet Radiol Ultrasound 2018;59(6):786–95.

2. Nolan MW, Gieger TL. Update in Veterinary Radiation Oncology: Focus on Stereotactic Radiation Therapy. Vet Clin North Am Small Anim Pract 2024;54(3): 559–75.

3. Nolan M, Elliott J. Neuro-oncology: radiation therapy and chemotherapy In: BSAVA Manual of Canine and Feline Neurology. British Small Animal Veterinary Association 2024.

4. Rohrer Bley C, Sumova A, Roos M, et al. Irradiation of brain tumors in dogs with neurologic disease. J Vet Intern Med 2005;19(6):849–54.

5. Körner M, Roos M, Meier VS, et al. Radiation therapy for intracranial tumors in cats with neurological signs. J Feline Med Surg 2019;21(8):765–71.

6. Brearley MJ, Jeffery ND, Phillips SM, et al. Hypofractionated radiation therapy of brain masses in dogs: a retrospective analysis of survival of 83 cases (1991-1996). J Vet Intern Med 1999;13(5):408–12.

7. Nolan MW, Dobson JM. The future of radiotherapy in small animals - should the fractions be coarse or fine? J Small Anim Pract 2018;59(9):521–30.

8. Schwarz P, Meier V, Soukup A, et al. Comparative evaluation of a novel, moderately hypofractionated radiation protocol in 56 dogs with symptomatic intracranial neoplasia. J Vet Intern Med 2018;32:2013–20.

9. Mariani CL, Schubert TA, House RA, et al. Frameless stereotactic radiosurgery for the treatment of primary intracranial tumours in dogs. Vet Comp Oncol 2015;13: 409–23.

10. Hu H, Barker A, Harcourt-Brown T, et al. Systematic review of brain tumour treatment in dogs. J Vet Intern Med 2015;29:1456–63.

11. Gieger T. Brain tumors. In: Plumb's Pro. 2022. Available at: https://app.plumbs.com/clinical-brief/2KXw7EzUg6VW9Ghn9n9Daf.

12. Ródenas S, Pumarola M, Gaitero L, et al. Magnetic resonance imaging findings in 40 dogs with histologically confirmed intracranial tumours. Vet J 2011;187(1): 85–91.

13. Troxel MT, Vite CH, Massicotte C, et al. Magnetic resonance imaging features of feline intracranial neoplasia: retrospective analysis of 46 cats. J Vet Intern Med 2004;18:176–89.

14. Axlund T, McGlasson M, Smith AN. Surgery alone or in combination with radiation therapy for treatment of intracranial meningiomas in dogs. J Am Vet Med Assoc 2002;221:1597–600.

15. Snyder JM, Lipitz L, Skorupski KA, et al. Secondary intracranial neoplasia in the dog: 177 cases. J Vet Intern Med 2008;22:172–7.

16. Toyoda I, Vernau W, Sturges BK, et al. Clinicopathological characteristics of histiocytic sarcoma affecting the central nervous system in dogs. J Vet Intern Med 2019;34:828–37.

17. Beckmann K, Carrera I, Steffen F, et al. A newly designed radiation therapy protocol in combination with prednisolone as treatment for meningoencephalitis of unknown origin in dogs: a prospective pilot study introducing magnetic resonance spectroscopy as monitor tool. Acta Vet Scand 2015;57:4.

18. Harzig R, Beckmann K, Korner M, et al. A shortened whole brain radiation therapy protocol for meningoencephalitis of unknown origin in dogs. Front Vet Sci 2023;10.

19. Monforte Monterio SR, Rossmeisel JH, Russell J, et al. Effect of radiotherapy on freedom from seizures in dogs with brain tumors. J Vet Intern Med 2020;84(2): 821–7.

20. Kelsey KL, Gieger TL, Nolan MW. Single fraction stereotactic radiation therapy (stereotactic radiosurgery) is a feasible method for treating intracranial meningiomas in dogs. Vet Radiol Ultrasound 2018;59(5):632–8.
21. Griffin LR, Nolan MW, Selmic LE, et al. Stereotactic radiation therapy for treatment of canine intracranial meningiomas. Vet Comp Oncol 2016;14:e158–70.
22. Snyder JM, Shofer FS, Van Winkle TJ, et al. Canine intracranial primary neoplasia: 173 cases. J Vet Intern Med 2006;20(3):669–75.
23. Hansen KS, Li CF, Theon AP, et al. Stereotactic radiotherapy outcomes for intraventricular brain tumours in 11 dogs. Vet Comp Oncol 2023;21(4):665–72.
24. Trageser E, Martin T, Burdekin B, et al. Efficacy of stereotactic radiation therapy for the treatment of confirmed or presumed canine glioma. Vet Comp Oncol 2023; 21(4):665–72.
25. Rohrer Bley C, Staudinger C, Bley T, et al. Canine presumed glial tumours treated with radiotherapy: is there an inferior outcome in tumours contacting the subventricular zone? Vet Comp Oncol 2022;20(1):29–34.
26. Dolera M, Malfassi L, Bianchi C, et al. Frameless stereotactic radiotherapy alone and combined with temozolomide for presumed canine gliomas. Vet Comp Oncol 2018;16(1):90–101.
27. Dolera M, Malfassi L, Marcarini S, et al. High dose hypofractionated frameless volumetric modulated arc radiotherapy is a feasible method for treating canine trigeminal nerve sheath tumors. Vet Radiol Ultrasound 2018;59(5):624–31.
28. Swift KE, McGrath S, Nolan MW, et al. Clinical and imaging findings, treatments, and outcomes in 27 dogs with imaging diagnosed trigeminal nerve sheath tumors: A multi-center study. Vet Radiol Ultrasound 2017;58(6):679–89.
29. Hansen KS, Zwingenberger AL, Theon AP, et al. Treatment of MRI-Diagnosed Trigeminal Peripheral Nerve Sheath Tumors by Stereotactic Radiotherapy in Dogs. J Vet Intern Med 2016;30(4):1112–20.
30. Sweet KA, Nolan MN, Yoshikawa H, et al. Stereotactic radiation therapy for canine multilobular osteochondrosarcoma: Eight cases. Vet Comp Oncol 2020;18:76–83.
31. Theon AP, Lecouteur RA, Carr EA, et al. Influence of tumour cell proliferation and sex-hormone receptors on effectiveness of radiation therapy for dogs with incompletely resected meningiomas. J Am Vet Med Assoc 2000;216(701–707):684–705.
32. Keyerleber MA, McEntee MC, Farrelly J, et al. Three-dimensional conformal radiation therapy alone or in combination with surgery for treatment of canine intracranial meningiomas. Vet Comp Oncol 2015;13:385–97.
33. Dolera M, Malfassi L, Pavesi S, et al. Stereotactic Volume Modulated Arc Radiotherapy in Canine Meningiomas: Imaging-Based and Clinical Neurological Posttreatment Evaluation. J Am Anim Hosp Assoc 2018;54(2):77–84.
34. Treggiari E, Maddox TW, Goncalves R, et al. Retrospective comparison of three-dimensional conformal radiation therapy vs. prednisolone alone in 30 cases of canine infratentorial brain tumours. Vet Radiol Ultrasound 2017;58:106–16.
35. Benedict SH, Yenice KM, Followill D, et al. Stereotactic body radiation therapy: the report of AAPM Task Group 101. Med Phys 2010;37(8):4078–101.
36. Rancilio NJ, Bentley RT, Plantenga JP, et al. Safety and feasibility of stereotactic radiotherapy using computed portal radiography for canine intracranial tumors. Vet Radiol Ultrasound 2018;59(2):212–20.
37. Rossmeisl JH, Jones JC, Zimmerman KL, et al. Survival time following hospital discharge in dogs with palliatively treated primary brain tumors. J Am Vet Med Assoc 2013;242(2):193–8.
38. Heidner GL, Kornegay JN, Page RL, et al. Analysis of survival in a retrospective study of 86 dogs with brain tumors. J Vet Intern Med 1991;5(4):219–26.

39. Moirano SJ, Dewey CW, Haney S, et al. Efficacy of frameless stereotactic radiotherapy for the treatment of presumptive canine gliomas. Vet Comp Oncol 2020; 18:528–37.
40. Nguyen SM, Thamm DM, Vail DM, et al. Response evaluation criteria for solid tumors in dogs (v1.0). Vet Comp Oncol 2013;13(3):176–83.
41. Camerson S, Rishniw M, Miller AD, et al. Characteristics and survival of 121 cats undergoing excision of intracranial meningiomas. Vet Surg 2015;44(6):772–6.
42. Tomek A, Cizinauskas S, Doherr M, et al. Intracranial neoplasia in 61 cats: localisation, tumour types and seizure patterns. J Feline Med Surg 2006;8(4):243–53.
43. Troxel MT, Vite CH, Van Winkle TJ, et al. Feline intracranial neoplasia: retrospective review of 160 cases (1985-2001). J Vet Intern Med 2003;17(6):850–9.
44. Westworth DR, Dickinson PJ, Vernau W, et al. Choroid plexus tumors in 56 dogs (1985-2007). J Vet Intern Med 2008;22(5):1157–65.
45. Brehm DM, Vite CH, Steinberg HS, et al. A retrospective evaluation of 51 cases of peripheral nerve sheath tumours in the dog. J Am Anim Hosp Assoc 1995;31: 349–59.
46. Holmes ME, Keyerleber MA, Faissler D. Prolonged survival after craniectomy with skull reconstruction and adjuvant definitive radiation therapy in three dogs with multilobular osteochondrosarcoma. Vet Radiol Ultrasound 2019;60:447–55.
47. Dernell WS, Straw RC, Cooper MF, et al. Multilobular osteochondrosarcoma in 39 dogs: 1979-1993. J Am Anim Hosp Assoc 1998;34:11–8.

Novel Treatments for Brain Tumors

John H. Rossmeisl, DVM, MS

KEYWORDS

- Blood–brain barrier • Glioma • Immunotherapy • Meningioma • Nanoparticles
- Oncolytic viruses

KEY POINTS

- The blood–brain barrier (BBB) and knowledge gaps in tumor biology remain significant obstacles to the development of effective treatments for brain tumors.
- Identification of shared molecular and genetic pathways that contribute to tumorigenesis in both dogs and people has been key to the discovery and translation of targeted pharmacologic and biologic therapies.
- Treatment approaches often utilize targeted or multifunctional antitumor agents, such as nanocarriers, molecularly targeted agents, immunotherapeutics, and oncolytic viruses in combination with alternative therapeutic delivery strategies that can overcome the limitations of the BBB.
- Many novel therapeutic strategies have been shown to be feasible, safe, or demonstrated preliminary evidence of efficacy in dogs with spontaneous brain tumors; however, none of the treatments discussed here are widely available or approved for clinical use.

INTRODUCTION

Brain tumors are a common etiology of neurologic morbidity and death in middle-aged to geriatric dogs and cats.[1,2] While numerous neuropathologically discrete brain tumor entities have been reported, a limited number of tumor types constitute most cases seen in clinical practice. Meningiomas, oligodendrogliomas, astrocytomas, ependymomas (in cats), and choroid plexus tumors (in dogs) account for approximately 80% to 90% of primary brain tumors in dogs and cats, and pituitary tumors, lymphomas, and hemangiosarcoma are the most common secondary brain tumors.[1,2]

Significant advances in the diagnosis and treatment of brain tumors have occurred in the past 3 decades. Veterinary neuro-oncology practice has evolved in large part due to the parallel development and more widespread availability of advanced neuroimaging techniques, which have subsequently been intimately incorporated into

Department of Small Animal Clinical Sciences, Veterinary and Comparative Neuro-oncology Laboratory, Virginia-Maryland College of Veterinary Medicine, Virginia Tech, 205 Duckpond Drive, Blacksburg, VA 24061, USA
E-mail address: jrossmei@vt.edu

Vet Clin Small Anim 55 (2025) 81–94
https://doi.org/10.1016/j.cvsm.2024.07.008   **vetsmall.theclinics.com**
0195-5616/25/© 2024 Elsevier Inc. All rights reserved, including those for text and data mining, AI training, and similar technologies.

neurosurgical and radiotherapeutic procedural workflows.[1,3] Despite these improvements, with few exceptions, current multimodality treatments do not provide cures for canine and feline brain tumors, and local disease recurrence and tumor progression continue to represent common and challenging management scenarios for veterinary clinicians.[1] Thus, there is a clinical need for new and effective brain tumor therapeutics.

A similar unmet clinical need exists in humans, where malignant brain tumors also represent aggressive and treatment-refractory cancers for which substantial improvements in survival have not been realized in decades.[4] The recognition that several types of naturally occurring canine brain tumors display similar clinicopathologic, neuroimaging, and molecular characteristics as their human counterparts has fueled the use of dogs as translational models in the therapeutic development process, with potential cross-species benefits to both humans and dogs with these difficult tumors.[1,3,5,6] The existing literature is heavily biased toward the use of tumor-bearing dogs as animal models for new treatment options for brain cancer, with no studies identified that formally investigate novel treatment options in cats with spontaneous brain tumors. While dozens of novel therapeutics have been evaluated in dogs with brain cancers, this article focuses on those studies published since the subject was last systematically reviewed in 2014.[3,5]

CHALLENGES TO AND OPPORTUNITIES FOR THE DEVELOPMENT OF BRAIN TUMOR THERAPEUTICS

Brain tumors present numerous challenges to the successful design and delivery of therapeutics. Notable obstacles include the presence of the blood–brain barrier (BBB) as well as knowledge limitations regarding the biology of tumors and their unique interactions with the brain microenvironment.[3–6] Many recent investigations have attempted to address and overcome aspects of each of these challenging areas with innovative, multimodality therapeutic approaches.

The Blood–Brain Barrier

The BBB represents the major physical and functional barrier that exists between the peripheral circulation and the extracellular fluid of the brain and is composed of specialized, non-fenestrated brain endothelial cells, a capillary basement membrane, pericytes, and astrocytic foot processes (**Fig. 1**).[6] Passive, diffusive transport across the BBB is limited to small, lipid-soluble and nonpolar molecules, with transcellular movement of polar ions, nutrients, and macromolecular complexes occurring via highly selective solute carrier systems or receptor-mediated or adsorptive-mediated transport processes.[6] Paracellular molecular transport across the intact BBB is prevented by the presence of tight junctions that exist between brain endothelial cells (see **Fig. 1**). Brain endothelial cell membranes also contain several families of drug efflux transporters that actively transport endogenous and exogenous compounds out of the brain endothelial cell cytoplasm.[6] While the selective permeability of the BBB serves an essential role in the maintenance of brain homeostasis and function, and protection from blood-borne toxins, it also prevents the majority of pharmacologic compounds from reaching therapeutically effective concentrations in the brain. Less than 5% of small molecule therapeutics effectively penetrate the BBB following systemic administration.[4–6] A major aspect of brain tumor therapeutic research revolves around developing compounds that are BBB penetrant or drug-delivery techniques that bypass the BBB.[1,3,5,6]

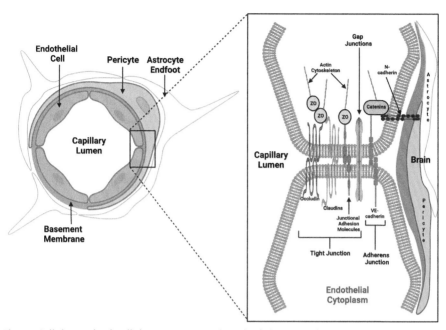

Fig. 1. Cellular and subcellular components (inset) of the BBB. The BBB is a structural and functional unit that includes brain endothelial cells, pericytes, astrocytic endfeet, and a basement membrane. Tight junctional complexes (inset) between endothelial cells restrict paracellular movement of substances across the BBB. (Figure modified from Partridge B, Eardley A, Morales BE, Campelo SN, Lorenzo MF, Mehta JN, Kani Y, Mora JKG, Campbell E-OY, Arena CB, Platt S, Mintz A, Shinn RL, Rylander CG, Debinski W, Davalos RV and Rossmeisl JH. Advancements in drug delivery methods for the treatment of brain disease. Front Vet Sci 2022; 9:1039745 (CC-BY); with permission.[6] Figure created with BioRender.com.)

Knowledge Gaps in Tumor Biology and Microenvironmental Interactions

Tremendous strides in the molecular, genetic, and epigenetic characterization of human brain tumors over the past 2 decades have resulted in major paradigm shifts in both the diagnostic approach to and prognoses associated with brain tumors.[7,8] Although numerous and relatively large "omic" datasets for multiple human brain tumor variants exist, there remain considerable knowledge gaps related to genotypic–phenotypic associations, as well as correlations that may exist between specific molecular aberrations and tumor clinical features. In veterinary medicine, classifications of tumor biologic behaviors and molecular landscapes are in their infancy, and prognostically relevant brain tumor morphologic or molecular alterations have yet to be identified.[9,10] However, cytogenetic profiling of canine brain tumors to date has identified several pharmacologically tractable and shared molecular alterations with human tumors, and some of these have been exploited to develop novel therapeutics with cross-species applications.[9,11,12]

Findings from the new but rapidly evolving field of cancer neuroscience have further illustrated the complexity and importance of interactions between cancer cells and the normal brain microenvironment. For example, certain types of high-grade gliomas are capable of integrating into neural networks through the formation of functional synapses between glioma cells and neurons.[13] Through these connections, tumors can hijack signaling pathways normally used for neuroglial development, communication, and plasticity to promote tumor growth and invasion.[13] These insights have identified novel mechanisms that could be targeted by repurposing drugs currently approved for other neurologic disorders, such as anticonvulsants, that were designed to modulate several of these tumor-promoting signaling networks.[13]

NOVEL BRAIN TUMOR THERAPEUTIC APPROACHES

Many of the treatments discussed here, either by necessity or for advantage, leverage the potential benefits of combining one or more novel therapeutic agent designs or delivery strategies.[3,5,6] For instance, the inherent biophysiochemical properties of many molecular targeted drugs, oncolytic viruses (OV), and immunotherapeutics render them incapable of penetrating the BBB when administered systemically.[1,6] Thus, these therapeutics require delivery by a method that bypasses or disrupts the BBB, such as direct intralesional injection, convection-enhanced delivery (CED), or focused ultrasound BBB permeabilization. Drug-delivery methodologies that have been utilized for the treatment of neurologic disorders in veterinary medicine have recently been reviewed.[6]

Passive Tumor Targeting

Passive targeting relies on a phenomenon common to solid tumors termed the enhanced permeability and retention (EPR) effect. The EPR describes the progressive entrance into and accumulation of macromolecular compounds within the interstitium of vascularized tumor regions.[14] Several pathophysiologic characteristics of solid tumors contribute to the EPR, including (1) the presence of extensive, but often structurally or functionally deficient, tumor neovasculature; (2) tumor elaboration of cytokines, such as bradykinin, vascular endothelial growth factor (VEGF), nitric oxide, interleukin-1 (IL-1), interleukin-2 (IL-2), interleukin-6 (IL-6), and prostaglandins, that directly or indirectly increase vascular permeability; and (3) impaired lymphatic drainage of tumor tissue.[14,15]

The design of nanotherapeutics seeks to further capitalize on the EPR effect by developing nanoparticles with specific physiochemical properties, such as size, surface charge, lipophilicity, and geometry in order to prolong drug circulation time as well as accumulation and persistence within the tumor interstitium.[15] It has been demonstrated that the ideal nanoparticular size range to enhance the EPR effect is 10 to 200 nm, and liposomal or polymer encapsulation of drugs is a commonly used approach to facilitate controlled drug release and the EPR effect, protect drugs from degradation and clearance, and minimize drug toxicities.[14] Several studies in dogs have utilized passively targeted nanomedical approaches to facilitate delivery of therapeutics to brain tumors.[16–18]

Arami and colleagues[16] utilized a deliver and resect study design to demonstrate the heterogeneity of the EPR effect in 4 dogs with intracranial meningiomas or oligodendrogliomas. In this study, PEGylated gold nanoparticles (GNPs) were administered intravenously 24 hours prior to planned tumor resection. The excised tumors were then analyzed using histopathology, Raman spectroscopy, mass spectroscopy, and scanning electron microscopy to document the presence of GNPs in various tumor microenvironmental (TME) compartments. While this study demonstrated that an EPR effect occurs in canine brain tumors, it also illustrated that the distribution of GNP was variable across tumor types, as well as within tumor regions, with no detectable GNP observed within necrotic tumor areas.[16]

Two studies have investigated intratumoral delivery of polymeric-controlled release formulations of temozolomide (TMZ) in dogs with gliomas, as this approach has been shown to increase cytotoxicity, decrease systemic drug-associated adverse events, and improve survival in rodent models of glioma.[17,18] Young and colleagues[17] performed a feasibility study whose primary endpoint was to demonstrate via MRI that polymeric magnetite nanoparticles encapsulating temozolomide (TMZ-NP) could be delivered intratumorally by CED. In this investigation, 10 dogs with presumed brain tumors received a single CED infusion, and the presence of TMZ-NP within the targeted region was confirmed in 70% of the cases using immediate post-infusion brain MRI.[17] Results of this study emphasize the need for incorporation of techniques that confirm agent delivery to the target when performing locoregional delivery techniques in the brain. The study design did not include systematic evaluations of antitumor effects of the TMZ-NP, as some enrolled dogs also received other treatments. Another study locally implanted biopolymeric microcylinders conjugated with TMZ and gadolinium into subtotally resected gliomas in 4 dogs.[18] The procedure was well tolerated in all dogs, and serial postimplantation brain MRI confirmed microcylinder placement and demonstrated further reductions in tumor volume compared to the immediate postoperative MRI in 2 out of 4 dogs.[18]

Nanomedical approaches have also been utilized to deliver radiotherapeutics to canine brain tumors. Pasciak and colleagues[19] treated 5 dogs with presumptive gliomas by trans-arterial radioembolization with Yttrium-90 (^{90}Y) microspheres. Immediately after treatment, the procedural technical success and dose distribution were determined via ^{90}Y positron emission tomography (PET)-CT, and the dogs were followed for 6 months with serial clinical and brain MRI examinations. Trans-arterial delivery of ^{90}Y to the lesion was achieved in all dogs in this study, although the vascular anatomy of the dogs precluded super-selective arterial radioembolizations.[19] One dog died within 24 hours of the procedure, and 3 out of 4 dogs that survived developed transient interictal neurologic deficits that were possibly attributed to microsphere-induced cerebral ischemic changes outside the intended target region due to nonselective arterial catheterization.[19] Reductions in MRI lesion volumes were observed in 4 dogs 1 month posttreatment. Another case report demonstrated the feasibility of utilizing holmium-166 brachytherapy in a dog with a pituitary macrotumor.[20] Stereotactic intratumoral injection of holmium-166 microspheres in this dog resulted in a 40% reduction in the tumor volume and transient improvement in neurologic signs.[20]

Active Tumor Targeting

Active targeting refers to ligand–receptor specific interactions between a drug or carrier and a target cell.[1,21] In the context of cancer therapy, targeted agents are typically designed to modulate signal transduction pathways involved in cell growth, proliferation, ephrins (EPH) and survival or promotion of antitumor immunity. Active targeting takes advantage of molecular, genetic, or epigenetic alterations that are exclusively present or differentially expressed in tumor cells or the TME compared to normal cells.[21] As a result, active targeting theoretically has more specific antitumor activity and less toxicity than conventional chemotherapeutics or passively targeted drugs. A significant limitation of targeted therapeutics is that the target of interest must be present in the tumor to realize the therapeutic effects, and this has many practical implications in veterinary medicine considering the infrequency with which brain tumors are biopsied prior to treatment.[1,11]

A diverse repertoire of targeted agents have been tested in early phase studies in dogs with brain tumors, with candidates consisting of recombinant bacterial cytotoxins, functionalized nanoparticles, immune-checkpoint inhibitors (ICI), and protease-targeted OV.[1,3,5,11,12,21–25] Although ICI and engineered OV are technically forms of targeted therapy, these are often classified as their own types of therapeutics and are reviewed separately.[24,25]

Several studies have exploited the overexpression of cell surface tyrosine kinase and cytokine receptors that occur on human and canine gliomas, including epidermal growth factor (EGFR), ephrins (EPH), and interleukin-13 receptor alpha 2 (IL-13RA2) (**Fig. 2**).[9,11,12,21,22] A canine phase I trial administered recombinant bacterial cytotoxins conjugated to IL-13RA2 and EPHA2 receptor ligands by imaging monitored CED to 17 dogs with intracranial gliomas that were confirmed to express these targets.[11] Tumors were successfully infused via CED in all dogs, and no dose-limiting toxicities occurred in any of the 6 escalating dose cohorts. A single cytotoxin treatment resulted in objective tumor responses, characterized by 65% or greater reductions in posttreatment MRI tumor volumes and improvements in clinical signs, in 50% of the dogs, including at least one dog in each of the 5 highest dosing cohorts.[11] This therapeutic approach has been expanded in an active canine clinical trial investigating single pharmaceutical agents (QUAD compounds) that are capable of simultaneously targeting IL13-RA2, EPHA2, EPHA3, and EPHB2 receptors, which are expressed in multiple glioma microenvironmental compartments (**Fig. 3**).[21]

Two studies have evaluated EGFR-targeted therapeutics in dogs with brain tumors.[12,23] Freeman and colleagues[12] treated 8 dogs with oligodendrogliomas with intratumoral cetuximab conjugated iron oxide nanoparticles (IONPs) delivered via CED. Cetuximab is an anti-EGFR (anti-erbB1) monoclonal antibody that prevents downstream signal transduction by inhibiting activation of the EGFR tyrosine kinase. The cetuximab-IONPs were delivered to all dogs as confirmed with immediate postoperative MRI, and no dogs developed serious adverse events associated with the treatment. Tumor volumetric reductions attributable to the cetuximab-IONPs therapy were observed in 7 out of 8 dogs 1 month following treatment, including at least one dog whose tumor did not express EGFR, suggesting that clinically relevant off-target effects may be associated with this therapy.[21] In a proof of concept trial, bacterially derived minicells were packaged with doxorubicin and targeted to EGFR using bispecific antibodies and administered by repeated intravenous (IV) injection to 17 dogs with a variety of brain tumors.[23] In vivo single-photon emission computed tomography

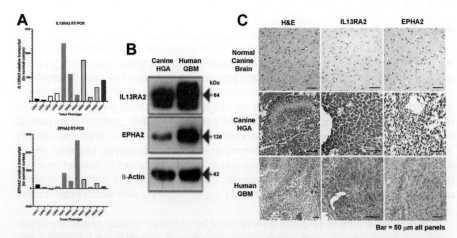

Fig. 2. IL13R-A2 and EPHA2 receptors are similarly overexpressed in canine (A, B, C) and human (B, C) gliomas, as demonstrated with gene expression (A), western blotting (B), and immunohistochemistry (C), with minimal expression in normal brain.[11,21,22] GBM, glioblastoma; LGA, low-grade astrocytoma; HGA, high-grade astrocytoma, LGO, low-grade oligodendroglioma; HGO, high-grade oligodendroglioma; HGU, high-grade undefined glioma.

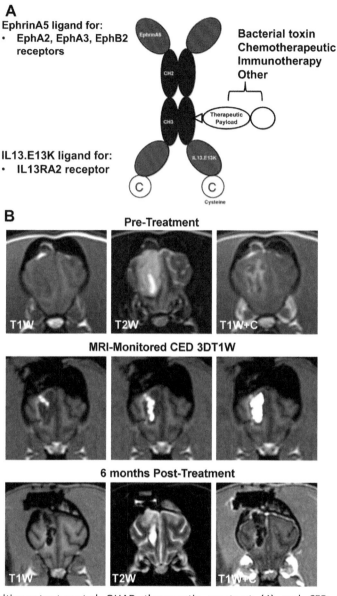

Fig. 3. Multireceptor-targeted QUAD therapeutic construct (*A*) and CED of QUAD-doxorubicin to a dog with high-grade astrocytoma expressing IL13-RA2, EPHA2, and EPHA3 (*B*). Top row (*B*) tumor features before treatment. Middle row (*B*) intraoperative MRI of CED treatment illustrating progressive coverage of the tumor with the QUAD, which is codelivered with galbumin to allow for quantification of delivery. Bottom row (*B*) the T2W and contrast-enhancing tumor burdens are markedly reduced after treatment, being replaced with a cystic, necrotic treatment cavity.

(SPECT) imaging demonstrated that Iodine 123 (^{123}I) radiolabeled minicells accumulated within canine tumors, and serial minicells infusions were associated with no significant toxicities. Durable and objective complete or partial tumor responses were seen in 4 out of 17 of the dogs, and an additional 10 dogs had stable disease.[23]

ONCOLYTIC VIRUSES

OV are wild type or genetically engineered viruses capable of infecting and selectively replicating within tumor cells.[25–30] Using OV for cancer treatment is often considered to be a form of immunotherapy, as OV possess multiple mechanisms of antitumor action (**Fig. 4**) including selective replication within and subsequent direct death and lysis of neoplastic cells, as well as induction of a systemic innate and adaptive antitumor immune responses.[26] The relative roles each of these mechanisms plays in the antitumor effect differ based on the type of cancer being treated, inherent characteristics of the specific viral vector, and complex interactions among the virus, the host's immune system, and the TME.

There are several potential advantages associated with the use of OV for brain cancer therapy. As OV are replication competent, the entire tumor burden does not necessarily need to be initially exposed to the virus.[26] Following infection of even a limited number of tumor cells, a substantial local bystander effect may be anticipated, whereby viral replication and release of viral particles upon cell lysis into the adjacent tumor occur with subsequent infection and propagation of virus in new tumor cells (see **Fig. 4**).[25,26] Further, this bystander effect may be amplified through the release of tumor neo-antigens following oncolytic cell death that promote a systemic adaptive

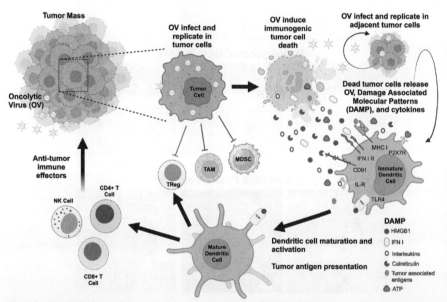

Fig. 4. Therapeutic mechanisms of oncolytic viruses (OV). Antineoplastic effects of OV occur directly through infection and lysis of tumor cells, as well as indirect facilitation of host antitumor immunity. Cellular lysis releases tumor-associated antigens and damage-associated molecular patterns, such as calreticulin, high mobility group box 1 (HMGB1), adenosine triphosphate (ATP), and cytokines that activate dendritic cells and stimulate an antitumor immune response. Natural killer (NK) cells and tumor antigen specific CD8+ cytotoxic and CD4+ helper T cells are the primary effector cells mediating antitumor immunity. OV may further alter the immunosuppressive tumor microenvironment by inhibiting (red brackets) functions of MDSC, TAM and regulatory T cells (Treg). CD, cluster of differentiation; IFN I R, type I interferon receptor; IL-R, interleukin receptor; MHC I, major histocompatibility complex Class I; P2X7R, purine 2 X7 receptor; TLR4, toll-like receptor 4. (Figure created with BioRender.com.)

immune response that has been shown in some preclinical models to be able to cause regression of distant tumor sites that were never exposed to the virus. Finally, certain OV vectors, such as Newcastle disease (NDV) and Zika viruses, are naturally neuro-tropic and capable of effectively crossing the BBB after systemic administration.[25,27]

There are also disadvantages associated with OV. The optimal dosing methods for OV are not established. As these are live viruses with proliferative capacity, there are challenges with pharmacologically modeling and defining effective doses, and there is a paucity of data associating the administered viral dose with in vivo replication effi-ciency or therapeutic efficacy.[25] OV that are not capable of penetrating the BBB require administration by local injection into the tumor or brain.[28,30] A better under-standing of the complex mechanisms involved in immune responses to OV is also necessary in order to balance the antitumor effects induced by antigen presentation and cytokine elaboration that occur during active viral infection against the develop-ment of neutralizing antiviral responses that inhibit viral replication and oncolysis.[25,26] There are also biosafety concerns associated with OV regarding potential transmis-sion of infectious virus to humans or animals in hospital or community environments.[25]

Wild-type Oncolytic Viruses for Canine Brain Tumors

Two dogs with intracranial meningiomas and one dog with an oligodendroglioma received therapy with intrathecal Brazilian Zika virus (ZIKV).[27] Although the authors stated no adverse events attributed to the ZIKV were observed, one dog developed presumed autoimmune encephalitis (leukoencephalopathy) after viral treatment that recurred upon subsequent viral rechallenge.[27] Improvement in neurologic signs occurred in all dogs following viral treatment, and serial brain MRI examinations ob-tained in 2 out of 3 dogs revealed potential tumor pseudoprogression with overall sta-ble tumor burdens for 78 to 120 days after the first viral injection.[27] Postmortem evaluations of the CNS from treated dogs demonstrated immunohistochemical evi-dence of ZIKV within neoplastic cells, while normal neurons were spared.

Oncolytic adenovirus (ICOCAV15) has been administered by direct intratumoral in-jection to a single dog with an incompletely resected intracranial hemangioma.[28] Serial reductions in tumor volume, as demonstrated with MRI, were observed following the viral treatment, with a partial tumor response observed at 1 year. A second dose of ICOCAV15 was administered upon identification of progressive tumor disease at 18 months, and the dog lived for an additional 13 months. No adverse effects directly attributable to ICOCAV15 were noted in this case. Comparisons of pretreatment tumor biopsies to samples obtained posttreatment and at necropsy revealed increased tumor-infiltrating B and T cells, and M1 macrophages following ICOCAV15 treatment, suggesting tumor immune activation.[28]

Engineered Oncolytic Viruses for Canine Brain Tumors

In a phase I/II trial, an engineered Lasota NDV strain targeting the urokinase plasmin-ogen activator system (rLAS-uPA) was administered by repetitive IV infusions to 20 dogs with a variety of intracranial tumors that expressed uPA receptor.[25] Dose-limiting toxicities manifesting as fever, hematologic, and neurologic adverse events occurred in 2 dogs. Mild, self-limiting adverse events, including infusion reactions, diarrhea, and fever, were common in dogs treated at or below the maximum tolerated dose (MTD). Partial tumor volumetric reductions occurred in 2 out of 11 dogs receiving the MTD, and the 3 month and 6 month progression-free survival fractions were 100% (9 out of 9 dogs) and 88% (7 out of 8 dogs), respectively for dogs in the Phase II arm of the trial.[25] Neutralizing antibodies to rLAS-uPA developed rapidly in all dogs, and viral genetic material was detectable in posttreatment tumor samples from 6 dogs.

Although systemically administered rLAS-uPA was well tolerated and capable of infecting tumors, strategies to evade host antiviral immunity are likely needed to optimize this OV approach.[25]

Cloquell and colleagues[29] treated 10 dogs with rostrotentorial gliomas with 8 weekly cycles of IV allogenic mesenchymal stem cells infected with the canine oncolytic adenovirus ICOCAV17 (dCelyvir). Treatment was well tolerated clinically and biochemically, with no documented serious adverse events. Seven dogs underwent serial follow-up clinical and MRI examinations, with 2 out of 7 demonstrating partial responses and 3 out of 7 stable disease at 2 months posttreatment. ICOCAV17 was detected in tumor tissue of 3 out of 9 dogs subjected to necropsy. These findings indicate that systemically administered dCelyvir is safe, capable of entering the brain, and may result in objective antitumor effects in dogs with gliomas.[29]

A phase I trial investigated the safety and tolerability of M032, an oncolytic herpes simplex virus-1 engineered to express interleukin-12, in 21 dogs with intracranial gliomas.[30] Following tumor resection, M032 was locally delivered via a catheter implanted in the resection cavity. No significant adverse events attributable to M032 or dose-limiting toxicities were observed in any of the 4 escalating dosing cohorts.[30] A subset of dogs underwent comparative analyses of peripheral blood, and pretreatment and posttreatment tumor samples using multiplex cytokine arrays, flow cytometric, immunohistochemical, and gene expression analyses. In the blood, M032 treatment resulted in CD4+ T-cell activation and modulation of interleukin-4 (IL-4) and interferon gamma (IFNγ) production in CD4+ and CD8+ T cells, and upregulation of multiple cytokines.[31] Treated tumors demonstrated transcriptional signatures consistent with activation of interferon signaling, lymphoid and myeloid cell activation, and T-cell and B-cell immune pathways, findings supporting modulation of the TME by M032.[31] An extension of this study is currently ongoing, in which the ICI indoximod is being added to the M032 virotherapy.[30]

IMMUNOTHERAPIES

Cancer immunotherapies (IT) comprise a broad array of mechanistic strategies whose common goal is to initiate, potentiate, or otherwise facilitate an antitumor host immune effector response.[3,5,32,33] Compared to results achieved in other cancers, IT for brain tumors has largely been disappointing.[3,4] Conventional wisdom regarding the brain being an immunologically privileged organ has shifted based on evidence illustrating the unique nature of immune responses, as well as the multiple, inherent resistance mechanisms to IT that exist in the brain.[5]

The majority of recent IT approaches for brain tumors in humans and dogs are designed to promote host antitumor T-cell responses.[4,24] In the TME of many types of human and canine brain tumors, myeloid cells comprise a significant proportion of immune cells.[4,8,9,27] In addition to the intended effects of inducing T-cell infiltration into brain tumors, T-cell-directed IT may initiate and perpetuate a cascade of counterbalancing pro-inflammatory events that recruit immunosuppressive myeloid cells to the TME. These immunosuppressive myeloid cells have phenotypic and functional similarities to those that are responsible for attenuating T-cell responses in chronic viral infections and thus may negate antitumor T-cell responses induced by dendritic cell or tumor lysate vaccinations. Given the role these myeloid cells play in mediating adaptive immune resistance in response to T-cell activation, newer IT approaches are emerging that specifically target the immunosuppressive TME.[32] Further elucidating the biology of these cells and the mechanisms by which they negatively regulate antitumor immune responses will likely be critical to inducing effective and durable therapeutic responses to IT in brain tumors.

Tumor production of the immune checkpoint inhibitor CD200 has been shown to suppress host antitumor immune responses through interactions with its inhibitory receptor (CD200R1) on antigen-presenting cells (APC).[24] In addition, CD200-like activation receptors (CD200R4) also exist on APC that have opposing functions to the CD200R1, which facilitate antigen presentation and antitumor immunity when stimulated. One study explored intradermal administration of a canine-specific CD200-like activation receptor peptide ligands (CD200AR-L) in 20 dogs with intracranial gliomas in conjunction with an autologous tumor lysate vaccination following surgical resection of the tumor.[24] Dogs that received combination tumor lysate and CD200AR-L experienced a significant overall survival (OS) benefit (median 12.7 months) compared to a historic control cohort of dogs that received tumor lysate only (median OS 6.3 months). Preliminary data from this study also suggest that soluble CD200 concentrations in blood may have value as a biomarker of the glioma burden. Canine-specific mechanistic data directly supporting modulation of the TME by either the tumor lysate or the CD200AR-L were not provided.[24]

The study by Ammons and colleagues[32] combined 2 novel methods of IT in 10 dogs with intracranial gliomas. Treatment involved modulation of the immunosuppressive TME associated with tumor-associated macrophages (TAM) and myeloid-derived suppressor cells (MDSC) in conjunction with allogenic anticancer stem cell vaccination (CSCV) to promote antitumor immunity. Daily oral treatment with off-the-shelf drugs losartan and propranolol, which inhibit monocyte migratory capacity and cause depletion of MDSCs, respectively, was utilized to modify the immunosuppressive TME, and dogs received CSCV via subcutaneous injection on a biweekly to monthly schedule. Clinical and MRI tumor responses and patient peripheral immune responses were serially monitored for 1 year.[32] Significant local or systemic toxicities were not observed, 2 out of 10 dogs experienced partial tumor responses, and 6 out of 10 dogs had durable stable disease. Dogs that developed measurable anticancer stem cell antibodies experienced prolonged survival (median OS, 500 days) when compared to dogs that did not generate antibody responses (median OS, 218 days).[32] Results of this study were promising regarding the feasibility, safety, and preliminary efficacy of a non-invasive combinatorial IT strategy that employs myeloid immunodepletion and CSCV vaccination, which may allow for treatment of surgically inaccessible tumors.

The stimulator of interferon genes (STING) protein functions as a sensor of cellular stress, particularly the presence of DNA in the cytoplasm.[33] Activation of STING promotes downstream signaling that induces transcription of type I interferons and inflammatory cytokines that promote innate antitumor immune responses. Five dogs with gliomas were treated via intratumoral injections of escalating doses of a small-molecule STING agonist. Injections were repeated after 4 to 6 weeks for a total of 2 treatments.[33] One dog experienced a serious procedural adverse event, characterized by a rapidly progressive local inflammatory response to the treatment, that resulted in euthanasia, and an MTD of 15 μg/injection was identified. In the 4 dogs in which post-treatment tumor responses could be evaluated, objective dose-dependent reductions in tumor volumes were observed, including one dog that experienced a complete tumor response following the second injection.[33] Results of this study were encouraging from the standpoints of the safety profile, relatively simple stereotactic method of delivery required, and the radiographic responses observed.

SUMMARY AND FUTURE DEVELOPMENTS

In dogs with naturally occurring brain tumors, multiple novel therapeutic strategies have been shown to be safe and feasible, demonstrated preliminary efficacy signals, contributed to the characterization of the mechanism of action of the tested therapeutic, or been translated for human indications. However, none of the treatments discussed here are available or approved for routine clinical use. Advancement of veterinary neuro-oncology, in the context of both conventional and investigational therapeutics, will require major practice paradigm shifts that recognize and embrace the need for histopathologic tumor diagnosis *prior* to treatment, as well as regular use of harmonized, objective, and clinically relevant therapeutic response and adverse event assessments, as are routinely done for other cancers[1,3,5] These practices will be fundamental to better characterize the natural history and biology of brain tumors, identify standard of care therapies (which are necessary for the assessment of relative risks and benefits offered by new treatments), and develop individualized patient management plans. In the current and coming ages of novel targeted-therapeutics and immunotherapeutics, the ability to define and compare the TME of naïve and treated tumors will be crucial for elucidating mechanisms of therapeutic efficacy and resistance, as well as selecting appropriate patients for treatment.[11,31] Comprehensive morphologic and molecular characterization of tumors has revolutionized the diagnostic and prognostic landscapes of human brain tumors.[7,8] Given the improvements in tools available for the molecular, genetic, and epigenetic analyses of veterinary brain tumors, adopting a similar approach will likely provide the greatest future opportunities for improving therapeutic outcomes, as well as identifying additional novel oncogenic pathways that could be exploited for the potential benefit of animals and humans with brain tumors.[9–11]

DISCLOSURE

J.H. Rossmeisl holds patents and has patents pending on QUAD compound targeted and oncolytic viral therapeutics for cancer and is an advisory board member with Zoetis.

FUNDING

Data appearing in portions of this manuscript were supported by NIH R21AI070528, NIH P01CA207206, NIH R01CA139099, and NIH R01CA276233 to JHR.

REFERENCES

1. Miller AD, Miller CR, Rossmeisl JH. Canine primary intracranial cancer: A clinicopathologic and comparative review of glioma, meningioma, and choroid plexus tumors. Front Oncol 2019;9:1151.
2. Troxel MT, Vite CH, Van Winkle TJ, et al. Feline intracranial neoplasia: retrospective review of 160 cases (1985-2001). J Vet Intern Med 2003;17(6):850–9.
3. Dickinson PJ. Advances in diagnostic and treatment modalities for intracranial tumors. J Vet Intern Med 2014;28(4):1165–85.
4. Schaff LR, Mellinghoff IK. Glioblastoma and other primary brain malignancies in adults: A review. JAMA 2023;329(7):574–87.
5. Rossmeisl JH. New treatment modalities for brain tumors in dogs and cats. Vet Clin North Am Small Anim Pract 2014;44(6):1013–38.
6. Partridge B, Eardley A, Morales BE, et al. Advancements in drug delivery methods for the treatment of brain disease. Front Vet Sci 2022;9:1039745.
7. Louis DN, Perry A, Wesseling P, et al. The 2021 WHO classification of tumors of the central nervous system: a summary. Neuro Oncol 2021;23:1231–51.

8. Cancer Genome Atlas Research Network. Comprehensive genomic characterization defines human glioblastoma genes and core pathways. Nature 2008; 455(7216):1061–8.
9. Amin SB, Anderson KJ, Boudreau CE, et al. Comparative molecular life history of spontaneous canine and human gliomas. Cancer Cell 2020;37(2):243–57.e7.
10. Zakimi N, Mazcko CN, Toedebusch C, et al. Canine meningiomas are comprised of 3 DNA methylation groups that resemble the molecular characteristics of human meningiomas. Acta Neuropathol 2024;147(1):43.
11. Rossmeisl JH, Herpai D, Quigley M, et al. Phase I trial of convection-enhanced delivery of IL13RA2 and EPHA2 receptor targeted cytotoxins in dogs with spontaneous intracranial gliomas. Neuro Oncol 2021;23(3):422–34.
12. Freeman AC, Platt SR, Holmes S, et al. Convection-enhanced delivery of cetuximab conjugated iron-oxide nanoparticles for treatment of spontaneous canine intracranial gliomas. J Neuro Oncol 2018;137(3):653–63.
13. Sprugnoli G, Golby AJ, Santarnecchi E. Newly discovered neuron-to-glioma communication: new noninvasive therapeutic opportunities on the horizon? Neuro-Onc Adv 2021;3:vdab018.
14. Hansen AE, Petersen AL, Henriksen JR, et al. Positron emission tomography based elucidation of the enhanced permeability and retention effect in dogs with cancer using copper-64 liposomes. ACS Nano 2015;9:6985–95.
15. Maeda H, Wu J, Sawa T, et al. Tumor vascular permeability and the EPR effect in macromolecular therapeutics: A review. J Contr Release 2000;65:271–84.
16. Arami H, Patel CB, Madsen SJ, et al. Nanomedicine for spontaneous brain tumors: A companion clinical trial. ACS Nano 2019;13(3):2858–69.
17. Young JS, Bernal G, Polster SP, et al. Convection-enhanced delivery of polymeric nanoparticles encapsulating chemotherapy in canines with spontaneous supratentorial tumors. World Neurosurg 2018;117:e698–704.
18. Hicks J, Platt S, Stewart G, et al. Intratumoral temozolomide in spontaneous canine gliomas: feasibility of a novel therapy using implanted microcylinders. Vet Med Sci 2019;5(1):5–18.
19. Pasciak AS, Manupipatpong S, Hui FK, et al. Yttrium-90 radioembolization as a possible new treatment for brain cancer: proof of concept and safety analysis in a canine model. EJNMMI Res 2020;10(1):96.
20. Morsink NC, Klaassen NJM, Meij BP, et al. Case Report: Radioactive holmium-166 microspheres for the intratumoral treatment of a canine pituitary tumor. Front Vet Sci 2021;8:748247.
21. Sharma P, Sonawane P, Herpai D, et al. Multireceptor targeting of glioblastoma. Neurooncol Adv 2020;2(1):vdaa107.
22. Debinski W, Dickinson P, Rossmeisl JH, et al. New agents for targeting of IL-13RA2 expressed in primary human and canine brain tumors. PLoS One 2013; 8(10):e77719.
23. MacDiarmid JA, Langova V, Bailey D, et al. Targeted doxorubicin delivery to brain tumors via minicells: Proof of principle using dogs with spontaneously occurring tumors as a model. PLoS One 2016;11(4):e0151832.
24. Olin MR, Ampudia-Mesias E, Pennell CA, et al. Treatment combining CD200 immune checkpoint inhibitor and tumor-lysate vaccination after surgery for pet dogs with high-grade glioma. Cancers 2019;11:137.
25. Rossmeisl JH, King JN, Robertson JL, et al. Phase I/II trial of urokinase plasminogen activator-targeted oncolytic Newcastle Disease Virus for canine intracranial tumors. Cancers 2024;16:564.

26. Sanchez D, Cesarman-Maus G, Amador-Molina A, et al. Oncolytic viruses for canine cancer treatment. Cancers 2018;10:404.

27. Kaid C, Madi RADS, Astray R, et al. Safety, tumor reduction, and clinical impact of Zika virus injection in dogs with advanced-stage brain tumors. Mol Ther 2020; 28(5):1276–86.

28. Delgado-Bonet P, Tomeo-Martín BD, Delgado-Bonet B, et al. Intracranial virotherapy for a canine hemangioma. Int J Mol Sci 2022;23(19):11677.

29. Cloquell A, Mateo I, Gambera S, et al. Systemic cellular viroimmunotherapy for canine high-grade gliomas. J Immunother Cancer 2022;10(12):e005669.

30. Omar NB, Bentley RT, Crossman DK, et al. Safety and interim survival data after intracranial administration of M032, a genetically engineered oncolytic HSV-1 expressing IL-12, in pet dogs with sporadic gliomas. Neurosurg Focus 2021; 50(2):E5.

31. Chambers MR, Foote JB, Bentley RT, et al. Evaluation of immunologic parameters in canine glioma patients treated with an oncolytic herpes virus. J Transl Genet Genom 2021;5(4):423–42.

32. Ammons DT, Guth A, Rozental AJ, et al. Reprogramming the canine glioma microenvironment with tumor vaccination plus oral losartan and propranolol induces objective responses. Cancer Res Commun 2022;2(12):1657–67.

33. Boudreau CE, Najem H, Ott M, et al. Intratumoral delivery of STING agonist results in clinical responses in canine glioblastoma. Clin Cancer Res 2021; 27(20):5528–35.

Transsphenoidal Surgery for Pituitary Tumors

Björn P. Meij, DVM, PhD, Lucinda L. van Stee, DVM*

KEYWORDS

- Pituitary neoplasia • Transsphenoidal hypophysectomy • Cushing acromegaly
- Neurosurgery • Cancer

KEY POINTS

- A multidisciplinary pituitary treatment team should include the surgeon, radiologist, anesthesiologist, endocrinologist, and intensive care specialist.
- Careful surgical planning based upon patients' skull characteristics and pituitary fossa anatomy remains the basis of transsphenoidal hypophysectomy, especially as complex skull anatomy may increase difficulty of approach, and successful removal of a pituitary mass, and may require additional surgical techniques.
- Standardized remission criteria for pituitary surgery are key in determining surgical success and to build confidence for involved veterinary professionals and owners.
- Standard monitoring after pituitary surgery should include endocrine testing for functional masses and/or repeat imaging for silent (nonfunctional) pituitary masses.
- The value of curative pituitary surgical therapy is still underestimated and training of professionals at the master level for pituitary adenoma surgery is needed.

 Video content accompanies this article at http://www.vetsmall.theclinics.com.

INTRODUCTION

Intrasellar masses often comprise pituitary neoplasms.[1,2] Pituitary tumors account for 13% of all intracranial tumors in dogs versus 9% in cats, and 10% to 17% in humans. In cats, somatotropic tumors are most commonly found, whereas in dogs, corticotropic masses are reported in the vast majority of cases.[1,3] Apart from endocrine active adenomas, and their rare counterpart adenocarcinomas,[1,2,4] there is probably a large proportion of unrecognized clinically nonfunctional adenomas (NFA) in dogs and cats that only become clinically evident when they exert a certain mass effect on surrounding brain structures leading to nonspecific clinical signs or more

Small Animal Surgery, Department of Clinical Sciences, Faculty of Veterinary Medicine, Utrecht University, Yalelaan 108, Utrecht 3584CM, The Netherlands
* Corresponding author.
E-mail address: L.L.vanStee@uu.nl

Vet Clin Small Anim 55 (2025) 95–118
https://doi.org/10.1016/j.cvsm.2024.07.009   **vetsmall.theclinics.com**

pronounced neurologic deficits.[5] In humans NFAs,[1,6] which are most commonly gonadotrophic adenomas, comprise more than half of all pituitary adenoma cases whereas in dogs and cats they are poorly recognized.[1] Most pituitary neoplasms originate from the adenohypophysis and may cause apoplexy.[7–10] However, non-neoplastic intrasellar masses may include Rathke's cleft cysts,[11] suprapituitary ependymal cysts,[12] and hypophysitis.[13,14] Other less common neoplastic masses reported in the pituitary gland and/or pituitary fossa include pituicytoma, ganglioglioma,[15] craniopharyngioma,[2] metastases,[16,17] or ingrowth of a different tumor like meningioma or granular cell tumor.[1,18] Secondary neoplasms within the pituitary gland have also been reported and include lymphoma, histiocytic sarcoma and malignant melanoma.[19] Transsphenoidal pituitary surgery may appear to be an invasive procedure for pituitary masses compared to other treatment options,[20–27] but it is the only treatment that provides a rapid removal of the neoplastic mass, ensures a definitive diagnosis, and can be a potential true cure in case of complete adenomectomy. While the transsphenoidal hypophysectomy procedure in dogs has been around since the 1950's, the procedure is still evolving. The value of 3D printed guides and high-resolution endoscopes to improve surgical outcome remains to be investigated. Patient follow-up and monitoring for recurrence will provide the evidence and information for further decision making. A standardized approach to follow-up should be implemented across borders.[6] (**Table 1**).

THE PREOPERATIVE PATIENT
Case Presentation: Endocrine versus Neurologic Signs

Case presentation can differ significantly between patients with intrasellar masses.[1–28] In endocrine active masses, the clinical signs often are seen early in the development of the mass. Hormone-secreting cell types of the adenohypophysis include corticotropic (Adreno-corticotropic hormone-ACTH-secretion), thyrotropic (Thyroid stimulating hormone-TSH-secretion), lactotropic (prolactin-PRL-secretion), somatotropic (Growth hormone-GH-secretion), and gonadotropic (Luteinizing hormone-LH-/Follicle stimulating hormone-FSH-secretion) cell types.[1] The most common types of endocrine active functional masses in dogs and cats include respectively corticotropic and somatotropic masses. Other functional masses that have been reported in dogs and cats include lactotroph (prolactin producing), plurihormonal and unknown types.[1] The most common clinical presentation with an endocrine functional pituitary mass is Cushing's disease (pituitary-dependent hypercortisolism, PDH) in dogs and hypersomatotropism in combination with uncontrollable diabetes mellitus in cats. Upon initial presentation to a surgeon, which is usually later than at the initial presentation to a referring veterinarian, most animals have received medical treatment for a substantial time (months to years). Long term medical treatment may predispose to larger pituitary masses due to the time factor but in case of corticotropic adenomas also due to prolonged lack of negative feedback inhibition on tumor tissue that may accelerate growth but also transition the biological nature of the adenoma to a more malignant invasive or carcinoma tumor type known as Nelson's syndrome in humans.[29]

Non-functional adenomas, which are silent tumors arising from the adenohypophysis, nonpituitary masses, metastatic/secondary tumors, and non-neoplastic masses usually present with neurologic signs. Neurologic signs include decreased mentation, blindness, and seizures[1,16,20–25,30–32] that may develop slowly over time but can also rapidly progress to severe central neurologic signs.[7–10] Speed of progression and severity of clinical signs mainly depend on the size of the mass and speed of mass development, and loss of the equilibrium between brain adaptation to incremental

Table 1
Standardized approach on follow-up and monitoring with respective challenges, considerations and future perspectives

	Time and Place	Challenges	Considerations and Future Perspectives
Pre-operative	Diagnosis	Location based differences in endocrine and imaging testing	Standardizing work up and implementing an international standardization among pituitary experts
	Surgical decision making	Predicting outcome due to the large variety of outcomes independent of pituitary pathology and pituitary size	Improved diagnostic imaging techniques, development and adoption of (bio) markers for outcome.
	Surgical planning	Increased size of pituitary masses presented for surgery	Strict monitoring of smaller pituitary masses with early intervention if growth is seen. Determining at what P/B ratio cut off surgical intervention is advised by data analysis, with or without the help of AI.
		Anatomically challenging cases	Use of 3D real time imaging and VR techniques. Prepare for additional interventions, if possible through simulation in silico. n
	Public ownership of patients?	Informing and reaching future clients through veterinary professionals and client groups on specific diseases like Cushing's disease (dog) and acromegaly (cat)	Stimulatig and supporting informed and experienced clients to form patient discussion groups on online forums or social media
Intraoperative	Navigation	Improving burr hole accuracy in a low morbidity and easily adoptable fashion	Compare different methods of facilitating the surgical approach in vitro and in vivo, with or without AI. Use of intraoperative real time imaging techniques like the Hololens.
	Visualization	Visualization of anatomic structures and residual tumor tissue within the fossa	Use of intraoperative endoscopy techniques vs real time 2D imaging methods like intraoperative MRI. Using different types of magnification or use of real time 3D and VR techniques.
			Use of intraoperative color coding of neoplastic tissue
	Teaching methods	Difficulty teaching approach and obtaining dexterity in vitro and in vivo	Using video assessment, 3D printing, in silico and VR techniques to teach the technique. Developing pituitary master courses by pituitary experts for training of surgeons

(continued on next page)

Table 1
(continued)

	Time and Place	Challenges	Considerations and Future Perspectives
Post operative	Inpatient management	Predicting intracranial complications, sodium imbalances and time needed for close monitoring. Breed specific complications in brachycephalic dogs Postoperative morbidity, mortality and prolonged hospitalization	Use of AI and deep learning to identify patient specific (bio) markers for such complications Proactive approach addressing BOAS prior to surgical intervention Using the knowledge and skills of endocrinologists and intensive care specialists by installing a multidisciplinary team for perioperative patient-specific care
	Monitoring outcome	Standardizing outcome parameters and assessment intervals Patient morbidity and mortality due to improper long-term management	International cooperation and data exchange Implementing a multidisciplinary approach for every step along the treatment route

Inspired from a table format from Kahn et al 2023(6)

increase in intracranial pressure. In hindsight, less obvious changes in behavior and nonspecific clinical signs including lethargy and inappetence may be present in the history, but are often overlooked or misinterpreted. A sudden onset of severe neurologic signs is seen related to sudden infarction and hemorrhaging in a pre-existent pituitary adenoma, causing a state of pituitary apoplexy which is considered a surgical emergency in humans.[7–10,33] Recently, a case report has described the surgical treatment of apoplexy in a dog.[8] In rare cases, an NFA is identified during an imaging procedure for non-related problems. These so called incidentalomas tend to be rather small and close monitoring may suffice. A study in which routine necropsies also evaluated pituitary glands in 136 dogs, 11 dogs had a pituitary corticotropic adenoma.[34] However, only 1 dog had clinical signs associated with the corticotropic mass.[34] The incidence of incidentalomas may be severely underreported.[1]

Diagnostic Testing

Endocrine testing

Pituitary endocrine disorders include hypercortisolism (96% in dogs and 23% in cats),[1,26] hypersomatotropism (71% in cats and 2 case reports in the dog),[1,35,36] and hyperprolactenemia.[37]

Endocrinological workup for Cushing's disease may include the ACTH stimulation test, low-dose (blood) or high-dose dexamethasone testing (urine cortisol creatine ratios [UCCR]) and/or basal plasma ACTH measurements.[26,38] Basal plasma ACTH and UCCR levels for Cushing's disease[38] can be used both preoperatively and in follow-up for monitoring remission. However, be aware of ectopic ACTH secretion by tumors outside the pituitary gland in a patient presenting with Cushing's syndrome.[39–41] In case of hypersomatotropism and diabetes mellitus, plasma Insulin-like growth factor-1 (IGF-1) and GH measurements can be performed whereas IGF-1 is considered the gold standard for diagnosis and monitoring remission after treatment.[42,43] Diabetes mellitus has also been described in a cat with a melanotrophic pituitary adenoma[44] and double pituitary adenoma.[45] There are no current reports on gonadotrophic or thyrotropic pituitary masses causing endocrine signs in dogs and cats. Primary hypothyroidism has been reported in conjunction with hyperadrenocorticism in 2 dogs,[46,47] of which once case showed a dual pituitary mass[46] and the other did not show pituitary masses on diagnostic imaging.[47] In human medicine, gonadotrophic pituitary masses releasing LH and FSH appear to be endocrinologically silent.[1] Pituitary masses removed in dogs and cats are not routinely tested by LH and FSH immunocytochemistry and therefore, the incidence of these tumors may be underestimated among non-functional masses.

In case of incidentalomas, or patients presenting with neurologic signs due to suspected non-functional pituitary neoplasia or non-pituitary sellar masses, endocrine testing can be performed[1,11,12,16,30–32] to investigate pituitary function, especially hypopituitarism. In small non-functional and non-clinical pituitary masses, monitoring can be advised.[48]

Imaging

In patients diagnosed with Cushing's syndrome, imaging should include both the pituitary and adrenal glands.[49] Ultrasonography may be sufficient for adrenal assessment, but contrast computed tomography (CT) or MRI is preferred for pituitary imaging.[50–52] In case of Cushing's disease, contrast enhanced CT is preferred in many locations because of speed of the study and can easily include the complete skull, neck, thorax, and abdomen for assessment of skull anatomy, pituitary size, airways, cardiopulmonary issues and adrenal sizes.

Both high field MRI and CT imaging can provide information on the extent of the pituitary mass, the relation with adjacent anatomic structures and enable planning of the surgical approach. MRI shows the intricate details of the pituitary mass and the surrounding soft tissues but dynamic contrast CT scan[50] will also provide information on the pituitary gland as it lies outside of the blood-brain barrier. In addition, CT will also provide detailed information on the osseous landmarks for the surgical approach.[52] However, specific details of the soft tissue components of the brain surrounding the pituitary may be lost to evaluation in the CT scan. Developments within diagnostic imaging modalities, like image fusion (CT and MRI) technology and synthetic CT (bone sequence derived from high field MRI) would be a great asset to the pituitary surgeon.[53]

Molecular imaging with PET/CT, expands the possibilities of regular imaging. There is a wide variety of tracers available, and the most commonly used oncologic tracer in veterinary medicine is 2-Deoxy-2-[^{18}F]fluoro-D-glucose, also known as ^{18}F-FDG or FDG.[54–58] Combining PET/CT and MRI can improve further visualization of active pituitary masses, for example, using the tracer 11C-methionine-PET.[59]

Case Selection Considerations

When considering a case for pituitary surgery, tumor size, anatomy of the skull, and comorbidities should be well evaluated to prevent perioperative complications and inadvertent recurrent or residual disease. Though complete excision is preferred in any oncologic procedure, in large pituitary masses the surgeon should consider a safer approach, in which a mass debulking procedure and sequential treatments are the goal.

Surgical anatomy

Skull anatomy plays an important role in the surgical planning of the transsphenoidal hypophysectomy procedure. In breeds with mesocephalic and dolichocephalic skull types, there is generally more space than in brachycephalic breeds. In some cases, the hamuloid processes are pointed medially and may need to be distracted to gain sufficient access to the sphenoid bone.

Generally, cats provide a wider nasopharynx compared to dogs, and due to their shorter skull and ability to open the mouth quite wide, the approach can appear to be easier. Also, the air-filled sphenoid sinus in cats helps in pituitary fossa localization and experienced pituitary surgeons feel that the surgery in cats is easier than in dogs. These benefits, however, are counteracted by the small size of the skull (**Fig. 1**).

Where cats, mesocephalic and dolichocephalic dogs generally allow a good access to the sphenoid bone, brachycephalic dogs may need some more considerations. When performing imaging of the pituitary mass, the hard palate and its caudal extension over the sphenoid bones should also be evaluated. In severe brachycephalic dogs, the hard palate often obscures the burr hole trajectory over a length of 1 to 2 cm. As this will complicate the approach, a CT scan for this area is recommended over only an MRI of the pituitary.[52] (**Fig. 2**).

In order to prevent upper airway obstruction in severe brachycephalic patients due to post-surgical swelling and subsequent temporary upper airway stenosis, the authors advice to address any brachycephalic obstructive airway syndrome (BOAS) related concerns at least 14 days prior to a transsphenoidal hypophysectomy.[52] The owner and the postoperative care team need to be informed and ready to perform any treatment necessary in case of upper airway blockage. Novel treatments for increasing nasopharyngeal airway passage, such as temporary stent placement in brachycephalic breeds may need to be developed to counter the effects of postoperative swelling and subsequent upper airway blockage and dyspnea.

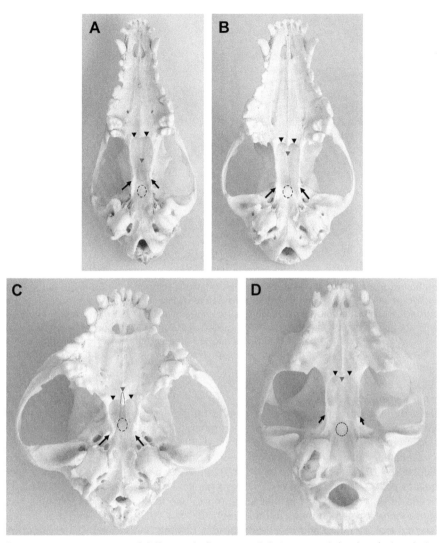

Fig. 1. Anatomic variation of different skull types and their anatomic landmarks in relation to the pituitary fossa. Direct ventral view of the skull base: (*A*) Dolichocephalic skull type, (*B*) Mesocephalic skull type, (*C*) Brachycephalic skull type, (*D*) Feline skull type. The distance between the caudal border of the hard palate (*black arrow heads*) and the rostral tip of the presphenoid bone (*red arrowhead*) is significantly different depending on skull type. The distance decreases with the relative shortening of the skull in the dog, with the rostral tip of the presphenoid bone even being obscured by the hard palate in brachycephalic dogs (*dotted line* image 1D). The pterygoid hamuli (*black arrows*) are easily palpable in the patient and their most caudal tip can also be used to estimate the location of the pituitary fossa (circle with dashed *line*). Depending on the skull type, the pituitary fossa can be caudal to the pterygoid hamuli (1D, cats and 1A, dolichocephalic dogs), at the level of the pterygoid hamuli (1B, mesocephalic dogs) and rostral to the pterygoid hamuli (1C, brachycephalic dogs).

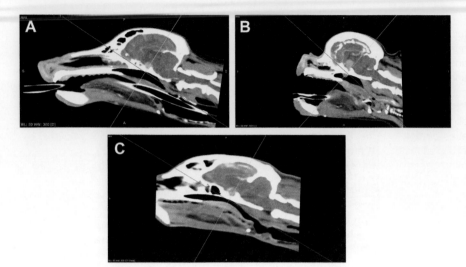

Fig. 2. Sagittal view of the approach within different skull types. (*A*) a normal skull of a mesocephalic dog. The end of the hard palate lies relatively rostral to the sphenoid bone. (*B*) a brachycephalic skull type, showing the hard palate in line of the view and obscuring the approach to the sphenoid bone. In general, distance from the end of the hard palate to the line of approach of the center of the pituitary fossa should measure at least 1,5 cm. If less, resection of the hard palate is necessary. (*C*) a feline patient showing the ample space within the oral cavity. Multiplanar reconstructions made in RadiAnt DICOM Viewer (Medixant).

Tumor anatomy and surgical intent

The size of the pituitary should be related to the size of the brain, as dogs and cats have a large range of skull sizes.[50,60] A normal pituitary in a healthy dog may range in size from 6 to 10 mm in length, 5 to 9 mm in width, and 4 to 6 mm in height. To classify a pituitary gland as enlarged, the pituitary height to brain area (P/B) value has to be calculated. P/B = height of pituitary (mm)/brain surface area (cm^2). A value below or equal to 0.31 is considered a normal sized pituitary, whereas any value above 0.31 is considered enlarged.[61] It is well accepted to use the terms macroadenoma and microadenoma when adhering to this threshold[61] but it must be realized that the human terminology micro and macroadenoma is defined on the 1 cm (10 mm) cut off value which cannot be extrapolated to the veterinary field. Unfortunately, the use of micro and macroadenoma terminology has created a lot of confusion especially in the veterinary radiological reporting. The use of the term macroadenoma should be used with caution since the implication of this terminology is a pituitary mass that has reached a considerable size with compression outside the fossa boundary on adjacent brain structures.

Besides the P/B value, a 5 point MRI grading system had been developed, determining the size and extension of pituitary masses, and correlating these parameters to outcome.[51] This is a useful tool that may also be extrapolated to CT imaging. Severe extension beyond the pituitary fossa often comes with displacement and/or obstruction of cerebrospinal fluid (CSF) flow in the third and lateral ventricles, and displacement or compression of the thalamus and optic chiasm. Decompression may improve clinical signs; however, chronic compression may have led to permanent damage and rapid decompression may lead to more damage through brain shift with concurrent complications.

Pituitary surgery with mass debulking can be a viable option for large and giant pituitary adenomas in dogs and cats with severe neurologic signs when no other treatment options are available.[12,30–32,51,62] The MRI grading system proposed by Sato and colleagues (2016) can give insight in the possible problems encountered during and after surgery in giant pituitary masses.[51] High grade tumors base on MRI and cases with a high P/B value (eg, > 1) will call for caution when proceeding for surgery. However, the authors and others[30,48] do emphasize that this should not exclude eligible cases for the transsphenoidal procedure. In selected cases, debulking or even complete removal of giant pituitary masses can be successful in the author's experience (**Fig. 3**). Informed consent, a well-trained team and planned postoperative management does need to be in place prior to any surgical intervention, especially in high risk cases like these. The post operative management can include ongoing medical management, with or without radiation therapy, follow-up imaging, and a second surgical excision.

The approach to the pituitary fossa can also be used to perform local treatments other than surgical excision. In a 2021 case report,[62] a pituitary macroadenoma was treated with injection of holmium spheres, providing a controlled and very local radiation treatment called [188]Ho microbrachytherapy. The case report describes a volume reduction of the mass of 40%, and a debulking surgery was performed at a later stage, when neurologic signs recurred. The scarcity of radionucleotides and the knowledge to manufacture carriers for these radioactive substances for local application, may provide the biggest hurdle in development of this therapy.

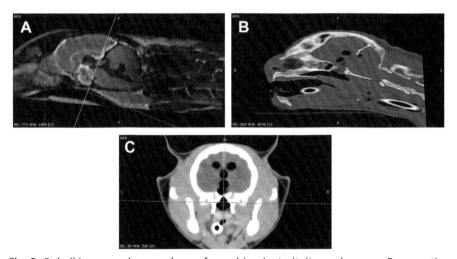

Fig. 3. Debulking procedure can be performed in giant pituitary adenomas. Preoperative imaging (*A*) and postoperative imaging (*B, C*) can be performed to assess completeness of excision. This is a case of a cat with apoplexy due to a silent pituitary adenoma and a severely enlarged pituitary gland. The preoperative MRI shows the extent of the mass (*A*). In giant pituitary masses, such preoperative imaging calls for a discussion with both owner and treatment team, to also plan for possible postoperative adjuvant therapies. Postoperative contrast computed tomography scan sagittal (*B*) and transverse (*C*) images shows no obvious signs of residual disease but will serve as a status quo to which follow-up imaging will be compared to. Multiplanar reconstructions made in RadiAnt DICOM Viewer (Medixant).

SURGERY
Anatomy Guided Techniques

Anatomy guided techniques will use intraoperative anatomic landmarks for orientation throughout the procedure as initially described by Meij and colleagues 1997 and later refined in 2001.[60,63,64] Anatomy of the individual patient and basic knowledge of the anatomic structures are essential for the approach. Intraoperative landmarks that are used for determination of the correct burr hole site in the preoperative imaging will help determine the exact relation of the pituitary fossa and the oral and nasopharyngeal structures that can be recognized during the surgical approach. All adaptations on the determination of the correct location for the burr hole do need this minimum data set for the surgeon to successfully perform the procedure. CT imaging and 3D skull reconstruction with DICOM software including a surgical knife software application will allow the pituitary surgeon to dry practice on the skull specimen in silico and practice the approach through the sphenoid bone and then check the location on the opposite site by removing the calvarium.[52] **(Fig. 4)** (Video 1) The surgical landmarks that need to be assessed on preoperative imaging are described in **Table 2**. These structures will guide the surgeon to the correct placement of the burr site without additional tools (see **Table 2**). (Video 2).

The current microsurgical approach was described in 1997,[63] however, modifications have been discussed in literature.[52,60,64,65] The authors have good experience with hypophysectomy using an operating loupe with 3.3 x magnification, with or without a head mounted surgical light, or just an overhead lighting. The operating loupe enables free rotation of the surgeon's head in all directions (similar to expensive freely movable floating neurosurgical microscopes) which is essential for neurosurgical procedures at the microsurgical level. In pituitary microsurgery the surgeon's view of the operating landscape should not be limited by the angular limitations of a magnifying device. (see Video 2).

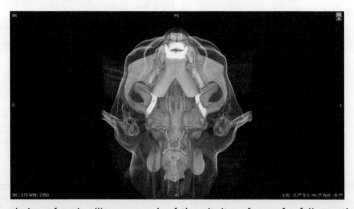

Fig. 4. Rendering of an in silico approach of the pituitary fossa of a feline patient. In an osseous window setting, all surrounding structures are removed digitally both ventral to the hamuloid processes and dorsal just above the tuberculum and dorsum sellae. The direct ventral view shows the undistorted view and the osseous suture lines of the presphenoid, basisphenoid and pterygoid bones. With the knife tool, a small pilot hole can be made, either from the dorsal side or the ventral side, to assess the exact location of the burr hole, and to relate this location to its intraoperative anatomic landmarks. The 3D reconstruction is made in RadiAnt DICOM Viewer (Medixant). Also see Video 1.

Table 2
Intraoperative anatomic landmarks for transsphenoidal hypophysectomy

	Anatomic Landmarks for Transsphenoidal Pituitary Surgery
Caudal tip hard palate	The hard palate is a palpable structure and the caudal tip can be easily palpated. On the sagittal multiplanar reconstruction with tilting of the skull base at a 40° angle like in surgical positioning, the distance between the end of the hard palate and the location of the pituitary fossa can be assessed and a distance of 1–2 cm enables an unobstructed passage through the soft palate to the pituitary fossa. In case of a distance of < 1 cm like in severely brachycephalic skulls, the hard palate overlays the sphenoid bones partially or completely. In these cases, a surgeon should plan and be comfortable and equipped to remove part of the hard palate during approach. This modification has been described by van Stee et al 2023.[52] An estimation of the portion that will need to be removed can be made when performing the approach in silico. In silico, the position of the skull should be rotated in the same position as the planned position of the maxilla on the positioning metal bar. Knowing upfront how far caudal the lowest point of the pituitary fossa is positioned in relation to the caudal edge of the hard palate, facilitates the approach through the soft palate.
Pterygoid hamulus	The left and right pterygoid hamulus are important landmarks for determining the location of the burr hole site. Depending on the skull type and reviewing the left and right pterygoid hamulus on the transverse spatial CT scan series, the pterygoid hamulus are level with the pituitary fossa (mesocephalic skull type), rostral to the fossa (dolichocephalic skull type) or caudal to the fossa (brachycephalic skull type). In silico, the position of the skull should be rotated in the same position as the planned position of the maxilla on the positioning metal bar. In some cases, the pterygoid hamulus deviate to the midline, encroaching the approach. Distraction of the pterygoid hamulus may be needed.
Craniopharyngeal pouch and duct	In some cases, a small or large fluid filled cyst like structure is present on the mucoperiosteal surface of the sphenoid bones [IMAGE pouches]. Almost always, careful eyescanning with magnification of the mucoperiost before incision, will reveal the 'birth mark' in the mucosa, a tiny whitish spot or fold which is a remnant of the trajectory of Rathke's pouch. This structure originates from the embryonic craniopharyngeal duct and was in direct contact with the pituitary fossa. In brachycephalic breeds this structure may reveal itself as a larger cystic pouch. The craniopharyngeal duct remnants, when removed, are sometimes also marked by a small blood vessel.

(continued on next page)

Table 2
(continued)

	Anatomic Landmarks for Transsphenoidal Pituitary Surgery
Intersphenoid and pterygosphenoid sutures	The pterygosphenoid sutures outline the presphenoid and basisphenoid bones on the lateral sides. The routine approach to the fossa is made in the basisphenoid bone and may extend somewhat into the presphenoid bone. The intersphenoid suture may not always be evident but lies just rostral to the emissary vein which protrudes in the most rostral part of the basisphenoid bone. This vein is not always evident.
Emissary vein	This vein originates from the craniopharyngeal duct and is often visible as a small bleeding hole in the basisphenoid bone.
Sphenoid midline	In the midline of the sphenoid bone, a ridge can be seen on the preoperative diagnostic imaging and can be palpated after the removal of the mucoperiosteum at the level of the presphenoid bone. Rostral to the burr hole site, the ridge projects ventrally, at the level of the burr hole site (basisphenoid bone), the ridge flattens out and caudal to the burr hole site, the midline forms a groove. The ridge is more pronounced in cats and may extend more caudally across the burr site than in dogs.
Cavernous sinuses	These sinuses can often be visualized when comparing the native CT or MRI and compare this to a contrast phase. Though these sinuses reside within the bone and encircle the pituitary fossa, they can cause significant hemorrhage during the approach. The osseous window often appears wider than the venous sinus is, and care should be taken not to damage the wall of the sinus.
Trajectory of the burr hole	The burr hole trajectory can be evaluated preoperatively using multiplanar reconstruction and 3D *in silico* techniques. Every association of anatomic landmarks with the trajectory can be identified preoperatively, and a plan can be drawn up to address any foreseen complicating factors.

Image Guided Surgery

Image guided surgery is a term used to describe a procedure in which the surgeon is using instruments to track their movements during a surgical procedure in relation to the patient, with the aid of imaging techniques.[66]

In 2018, a cadaveric study assessed the use of the Brainsight neuronavigation system (Rogue Research, Montreal, Canada) in the approach to the pituitary fossa. The Brainsight system has a widespread use in human neurosurgery, with a reported accuracy of 1.79 mm.[67] The median target error found in this study was 3.533 mm, though still within safety margins.[67] Main reasons given for the unexpected high target error, included errors in placement, registration, planning, scanning and burring. The true margin of error of the system is probably lower than measured.[67] Improved technique, practice, and the ongoing development of more sensitive systems should increase patient application and improve outcome in future studies.

Patient Specific Three-dimensional (3D) Printed Guides

With the increased availability of additive manufacturing, development and application of 3D printed drill guides have also been introduced in veterinary transsphenoidal hypophysectomy procedures. In 2 separate studies, the use of patient specific 3D printed drill guides to facilitate correct burr hole placement in transsphenoidal hypophysectomy in dogs was assessed.[68,69] Both studies encompassed both a cadaveric study and a small case series. The reported margin of error to the target location ranged from less than 0.1 mm to 0.46 mm (range 0–1.58 mm). The authors of both studies deemed the overall safety and efficacy of the procedure good.

Exoscopy and Endoscopy

Used as a magnification and lighting tool outside (exoscopy) and inside (endoscopy) the pituitary fossa, these techniques can aid in providing a better view of the approach, understand the anatomic details, and offer an additional educational opportunity to evaluate the technique and understand possible complications as video equipment offer the possibility of recording the procedure.

In order to improve intraoperative visualization, Mamelak and colleagues (2014) reported the use of a high definition video endoscope (VITOM^{tm}).[65] The set up has been a standardized method for this team and has been described in their 2017 review on transsphenoidal surgery for sellar masses.[48] The reported outcome is similar to that of the traditional technique.[48,65] Exoscopy can be considered a substitute to surgical loupes as described in earlier publications.[52,63]

During the last decade the endoscope has been used more and more and replaced the neurosurgical microscope in humans and made the pituitary surgery through the nose purely an endoscopic procedure.[70–73] The anatomic difference between humans with an air filled sphenoid sinus anterior to the pituitary gland, versus a bony wall between nasopharynx and fossa in dogs and cats, has limited the use of the transnasal endoscopic approach to the pituitary fossa in veterinary medicine. However, video endoscopy has been reported occasionally in transsphenoidal hypophysectomy procedures in dogs[52,74,75] and in case reports,[12,76] though descriptions lack technical details. After entrance to the fossa has been achieved in a transsphenoidal approach, a handheld video endoscope can aid in assessing the pituitary fossa when using an angled endoscope of at least 30° (**Fig. 5**). In the authors experience, in addition to a surgical loupe, video-endoscopy improves visualization, especially for assessment of structures within the fossa, lateral and rostral/caudal to the burr hole. Remnant

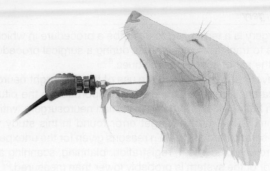

Fig. 5. Use of a hand-held videoendoscope. With a small diameter rigid endoscope, entry of the pituitary fossa can be achieved in the majority of cases. (*Courtesy* Remco van Deijk.)

tumor tissue that is beyond the visual field of the loupe or exoscope can be visualized, thus facilitating complete tumor excision.

THE POST-SURGICAL PATIENT
Clinical Outcome

Clinical outcome is the key measurement for effectiveness of a therapy. Over time, pituitary masses in dogs that are referred for surgical excision have increased in size.[38,52] Through improved preoperative diagnostic imaging, extensive surgical experience with different pituitary mass sizes in varying skull types, improved intraoperative visualization and dedicated post operative management, pituitary surgery in more challenging cases is also accommodated (**Fig. 6**).

Imperative for a good outcome is a well-organized intensive care with ample experience in dealing with patients post hypophysectomy. For the long term follow-up, management of the endocrine disorders created by hypophysectomy, should be in the hands of experienced endocrinologists. Comprehensive management of pituitary tumors includes pituitary surgery, radiotherapy and medical management.

Immediate postoperative intensive care

Hypophysectomy patients will need to be closely monitored for at least the first 24 to 48 hours. Patients with massive changes in intracranial pressure, cases with severe

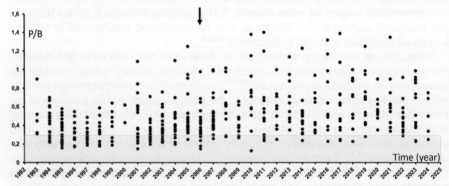

Fig. 6. Over time, the median size of pituitary masses has increased. Especially from the introduction of trilostane for the treatment of PDH (*arrow*), the pituitary size of patients receiving transsphenoidal surgery at our facility has significantly increased. The green line represents the 0.31 P/B ratio Year on X-axis, Size in cm on Y-axis.

neurologic changes, comorbidities like BOAS and cats with acromegaly and diabetes mellitus (DM) tend to need more time to stabilize after surgery.[5,8,31,32,38,42,43,52] Dogs with Cushing's disease tend to remain on the intensive care for a median time of 2 to 3 days[34,41] whereas cats with hypersomatotropism tend to need a longer time to be regulated in their salt and glucose homeostasis with a range of 3 to 21 days.[42,43] Animals with very large pituitary masses can do really well after decompression or do really poorly.[38,51] Overall, morbidity and mortality rises with increased size of the pituitary lesion[5,38,51,74] and the reported perioperative mortality ranges from 4% − 19%.

Intensive care and close monitoring remain essential. The minimal clinical data set in postoperative hypophysectomy cases should include serum sodium & potassium, urine production, fluid balance, temperature, bodyweight, ACTH in cases with corticotropic masses and blood glucose and IGF-1 in cases with somatrotropic masses.[38,42,43,60,63,64] If there are problems with mentation and intracranial pressures around the surgical procedure, an arterial line with continuous invasive blood pressure measurment should be instituted to titrate medication for treatment of a Cushing reflex.

Short term follow-up

Aftercare includes hormone substitution because of loss of pituitary function, and monitoring for ophthalmologic and upper respiratory complications.[60,63] The development of keratoconjunctivitis sicca after hypophysectomy is well recognized[38,42,43,52,60,63,74] and although it appears that the complication rate decreases with the surgical learning curve, it remains a clinical point of attention. Factors that negatively affect the tear production are brachycephaly, older age, endocrine disease in general, and anesthesia events. Al these factors contribute to the occurrence of dry eyes immediately following pituitary surgery.

Upper respiratory complications include rhinitis and soft palate dehiscence. Rhinitis is often transient and consists mostly of rhinorrhea and increased upper respiratory noise. In most cases, no treatment is necessary. Soft palate dehiscence is overall rare in dogs but may be more prevalent in brachycephalic patients in which the hard palate is also shortened. Soft palate dehiscence is more common in cats,[43] with a reported incidence of 8%,[43] and is associated with abundant use of electrocautery which should be avoided.

Long term follow-up

Lifelong supplementation with L-thyroxine and glucocorticosteroids require regular checks. In general, most patients will only need vasopressin supplementation for approximately 3 to 5 weeks, but some animals may remain dependent for months to years.[38,42,43]

For monitoring long term postoperative success in endocrine masses, follow-up should include regular monitoring of endocrine parameters linked to the initial pathology. In case of corticotropic masses, basal plasma ACTH levels, low dose dexamethasone suppression test or basal UCCRs can be done. In somatotrophic masses, IGF-1 measurement is needed to monitor remission. Initial endocrine tests are advised at 6 to 12 weeks postoperatively, every 3 months throughout the first year and yearly thereafter. In case of recurrence or residual disease, the testing interval should be adapted to the severity of clinical signs; pituitary imaging repeated and adjunctive treatment may be considered. There is a need for international standards for remission criteria in functional and nonfunctional pituitary adenomas. The authors propose a guideline in **Table 3**. In silent pituitary masses, follow-up should consist of repeat diagnostic imaging, with the first recheck at 3 months post surgery (see **Table 3**).

Table 3
Algorithm for diagnosis, treatment and follow-up

Parameters	Functional Pituitary Adenomas		Nonfunctional Pituitary Adenomas
Adenoma type	Corticotropic	Somatotropic	Gonadotrophic, Inactive hormone or subunit producing adenoma
Endocrine syndrome	Cushing's disease	Hypersomatotropism Insulin resistant diabetes mellitus	None, hypopituitarism, diabetes insipidus
Species	Primarily dogs, rare in cats	Primarily cats, rare in dogs	Dogs and cats
Diagnosis	ACTH stimulation LDDST, HDDST UCCRs, basal ACTH Pituitary imaging (CT, MRI) Adrenal imaging	IGF-1, (GH) Pituitary imaging (CT, MRI)	Pituitary imaging (CT, high field MRI)
Peri-operative monitoring (in hospital)	Plasma ACTH (pre-op, 1,3, 5 h post op) Immediate post op CT	Plasma GH (pre-op, 1,3, 5 h post op) Immediate post op CT	Immediate post op CT
Follow-up monitoring (home, > 2 wk post op)	UCCR (2 samples at home; 2 wk, 8 wk, 6 mo, 1 y, every year postoperatively) Imaging in case of recurrence	IGF-1 (GH) Imaging in case of recurrence	Imaging (CT, high field MRI) at 3 mo post op and then yearly

Abbreviations: ACTH, adrenocorticotropic hormone; reference after hypophysectomy preferably less than 5; GH, growth hormone; reference 39 to 590 µg/L; hr, hour; IGF-1, insulin growth factor-1; reference less than 1000 ng/L; reference after hypophysectomy preferably less than 50 ng/L; mo, month; UCCR, urine cortisol creatinine ratios; reference less than 10 x 10-6; after hypophysectomy values preferably less than 1 x 10-6; wk, week; yr, year.

Follow-up through diagnostic imaging should be performed on a case-by-case selection. If residual disease is present, postoperative imaging is advised. If the pituitary mass was non-functional and larger than the average endocrine functional pituitary mass[5] residual tumor tissue is more likely. Depending on size and type of mass, sequential imaging consisting of CT or MRI, should be performed around 3 months post surgery.

Histologic Outcome

The advantage of pituitary surgery is that histology and immunohistochemistry of pituitary specimens will confirm the nature of the pituitary pathology. There is a need for a standardized pituitary pathology protocol which includes immunostaining for a complete pituitary hormone panel. This will lead to a better understanding of NFAs, hyperplasia and incidentalomas. A recent report on pituitary masses in dogs and cats highlights the difference between veterinary and human medicine and exposes some of the gaps in our knowledge.[1]

CHALLENGES AND FUTURE DEVELOPMENTS

Pituitary surgery is becoming a more established surgical technique for the treatment of pituitary disease. Though the benefits of surgical excision of pituitary masses are a histopathological diagnosis, mass reduction, and complete resolution of clinical signs in many cases, hypophysectomy is costly, invasive and not readily available for the majority of patients. Radiation therapy is more available but often lacks resolution of endocrinological disease, and although medication may alleviate endocrinological disturbances, it will not prevent the mass from growing further and leads to inadvertent changes to the homeostasis. Combined therapies and pharmacologic developments may improve non-surgical outcomes.[21–27] However, hypophysectomy will remain a mainstay in the treatment of pituitary disease because it is the only curative treatment in functional pituitary adenomas as evidenced by full remission of endocrine hyperfunction and complete absence of pituitary tissue on imaging in case of nonfunctional pituitary adenomas. The challenges and future considerations are listed in **Table 1**.

Larger Masses and Challenging Cases Going Forward

The trend of patients presenting for transsphenoidal hypophysectomy with increasing size of pituitary masses over time has been noted in several studies. There are significant challenges that come with resection of larger masses[6,38,52,70–72] including intraoperative complications, a high chance of incomplete resection necessitating adjuvant therapy or repeat surgery, and persistent versus recurrent disease. Early detection and early surgical intervention have been advocated by several studies[52,77] to improve patient outcome. Though cases with non-functional masses that present once there are neurologic signs may not be detected early enough, small functional pituitary masses may be managed medically for too long, losing the window of opportunity of a surgery with less morbidity.

There is a role for each treatment modality and the choice of therapy should be tailored to the individual patient. In older patients, with a relatively small mass, opting for a medical management of their endocrine disease may be a reasonable choice. In younger patients, a more aggressive treatment may provide a better outcome in the long term. With the introduction of radiation therapy and drugs like trilostane for Cushing's disease, the value of surgery may be underestimated. However, radiation therapy does not cure the endocrine disease in functional pituitary masses and trilostane will not stop a pituitary mass from growing larger over time.

Improving Outcome by Measuring Surgical Success During and After the Procedure

There is not a standardized consensus on follow-up of pituitary pathology treated by hypophysectomy. The authors propose that surgical success of a transsphenoidal hypophysectomy should be investigated in a multimodal fashion. If applicable, endocrinologic testing may be the cheapest and most reliable technique in endocrine pathology (see **Table 3**).

Direct postoperative ACTH measurements in Cushing's disease are a good marker for complete or incomplete resection. However, endocrine testing is only performed once the procedure is finished. Intraoperative measurements of success currently mainly rely on solid surgical preparation, and visualization. Improved visualization can be achieved by advanced intraoperative imaging,[78] using fluorescent or tissue specific dies,[66,79–81] or even AR/VR.[82–88] Intraoperative success also largely depends on surgical dexterity that can be achieved in more ways than just by cadaveric sessions and clinical patients. For example, using AR/VR, practicing on life like 3D-printed mock ups,[89–92] AI and deep learning can help in surgical decision making.[93–96]

RECOMMENDATIONS

The authors call for standardizing work up and follow-up and working together on improving data collection and data sharing. More data may help develop more patient specific care and improve outcome.

Translational medicine can help our field forward. By borrowing and improving trailed and proven methods in human medicine for use in our small animal patients, we can benefit from their experience and efforts, while not endangering our patients with experimental techniques. Especially by practicing the surgery in progressively life like simulations and in vitro models, we can develop, improve and maintain dexterity without the ethical discussions of in vivo and ex vivo practice, and with a higher amount of repeatability.

In order to provide the best care, a multimodal approach to work up, surgery and postoperative care should be applied. Addressing each challenge together, with the shared knowledge and experience from specialists in their particular fields, will create a safe environment for all participants in the treatment team. Internal medicine, radiology, critical care, anesthesia and surgery are all essential disciplines that need to be involved to ensure the best outcome.

CLINICS CARE POINTS

- Pituitary neoplasia should be approached as a multi-disciplinary disease, where the combined efforts of internal medicine, imaging, surgery, neurology, and critical care specialists can bring the patient outcome to a higher level.

- Post operative critical care after transsphenoidal surgery is paramount for a good outcome.

- Cats with acromegaly and concurrent DM have an excellent outcome after pituitary surgery.

- Pituitary surgery remains a stable treatment option for a wide variety of patients as the quest for successful causative pharmacological treatments of pituitary disease is ongoing.

- Comprehensive management of pituitary neoplasia includes transsphenoidal surgery, adjunctive radiation therapy, medical management and/or repeat surgery.

DISCLOSURE

The authors have nothing to disclose.

SUPPLEMENTARY DATA

Supplementary data to this article can be found online at https://doi.org/10.1016/j.cvsm.2024.07.009.

REFERENCES

1. Sanders K, Galac S, Meij BP. Pituitary tumour types in dogs and cats. Vet J 2021; 270:105623.
2. Rissi DR. A retrospective study of skull base neoplasia in 42 dogs. J Vet Diagn Invest 2015;27(6):743–8.
3. Miller MA, Bruyette DS, Scott-Moncrieff JC, et al. Histopathologic findings in canine pituitary glands. Vet Pathol 2018;55(6):871–9. https://doi.org/10.1177/0300985818766211.

4. Nakaichi M, Iseri T, Horikirizono H, et al. Clinical features and their course of pituitary carcinoma with distant metastasis in a dog. J Vet Med Sci 2020;82(11): 1671–5. https://doi.org/10.1292/jvms.20-0500.
5. Hyde BR, Martin LG, Chen AV, et al. Clinical characteristics and outcome in 15 dogs treated with transsphenoidal hypophysectomy for nonfunctional sellar masses. Vet Surg 2023;52:69–80.
6. Kahn DZ, Hanrahan JG, Baldeweg SE, et al. Current and future advances in surgical therapy for pituitary adenoma. Endocr Rev 2023;44:947–59.
7. Woelfel CW, Mariani CL, Nolan MW, et al. Presumed pituitary apoplexy in 26 dogs: clinical findings, treatments and outcomes. J Vet Intern Med 2023;37:1119–28.
8. Tanaka S, Suzuki S, Oishi M, et al. Adrenocorticotropic hormone-producing pituitary adenoma with pituitary apoplexy treated by surgical decompression: a case report. BMC Vet Res 2022;18:397.
9. Galli G, Bertolini G, Dalla Serra G, et al. Suspected pituitary apoplexia: Clinical presentation, diagnostic imaging findings and outcome in 19 dogs. Vet Sci 2022;9:191.
10. Bertolini G, Rossetti E, Caldin M. Pituitary apoplexy-like disease in 4 dogs. J Vet Intern Med 2007;21:1251–7.
11. Van Blokland-Post K, Grinwis G, Tellegen A, et al. Transsphenoidal hypophysectomy as a treatment of Rathke's cleft cyst in a dog. Vet Rec Case Rep 2022;10:e427.
12. Lehner L, Garamvölgyi R, Jakab C, et al. A recurrent suprapituitary ependymal cyst managed by endoscopy-assisted transsphenoidal surgery in a canine: a case report. Front Vet Sci 2019;6:112.
13. Meij BP, Voorhout G, Gerritsen RJ, et al. Lymphocytic hypophysitis in a dog in a dog with diabetes insipidus. J Comp Pathol 2012;147:503–7. https://doi.org/10.1016/j.jcpa.2012.04.006.
14. Rzechorzek NM, Liuti T, Stalin C, et al. Restored vision in a young dog following corticosteroid treatment of presumptive hypophysitis. BMC Vet Res 2017;13:63.
15. Ishino H, Takekoshi S, Teshima T, et al. Hyperadrenocorticism caused by a pituitary ganglioglioma in a dog. Vet Pathol 2019;56(4):609–13. https://doi.org/10.1177/0300985819829530.
16. Gutierrez-Quintana R, Carrera I, Dobromylskyi M, et al. Pituitary metastasis of pancreatic origin in a dog presenting with acute-onset blindness. J Am Anim Hosp Assoc 2013;49:403–6. https://doi.org/10.5326/JAAHA-MS-5926.
17. Tamura S, Tamura Y, Suzuoka N, et al. Multiple metastases of thyroid cancer in the cranium and pituitary gland in two dogs. J Small Anim Pract 2007;48:237–9.
18. Barnhart KF, Edwards JF, Storts RW. Symptomatic granular cell tumor involving the pituitary glandin a dog: a case report and review of literature. Vet Pathol 2001;38:332–6.
19. Snyder JM, Lipitz L, Skorupski KA, et al. Secondary intracranial neoplasia in the dog: 177 cases (1986-2003). J Vet Intern Med 2008;22:172–7.
20. Schofield I, Brodbelt DC, Wilson ARL, et al. Survival analysis of 219 dogs with hyperadrenocorticism attending primary care practice in England. Vet Rec 2020; 186(11):333–60. https://doi.org/10.1136/vetrec-2018-105159.
21. Rapastella S, Morabito S, Sharman M, et al. Effect of pituitary-dependent hypercortisolism on the survival of dogs treated with radiotherapy for pituitary macroadenomas. J Vet Intern Med 2023;37:1331–40. https://doi.org/10.1111/jvim.16724.
22. Kent MS, Bommarito D, Feldman E, et al. Survival, neurologic response, and prognostic factors in dogs with pituitary masses treated with radiation therapy and untreated dogs. J Vet Intern Med 2007;21:1027–33.

23. Sawada H, Mori A, Lee P, et al. Pituitary size alteration and adverse effects of radiation therapy performed in 9 dogs with pituitary-dependent hypercortisolism. Res Vet Sci 2018;118:19–26.

24. Goossens MMC, Feldman EC, Theon AP, et al. Efficacy of cobalt 60 radiotherapy in dogs with pituitary-dependent hyperadrenocorticism. J Am Vet Med Assoc 1998;212:374–6.

25. Hansen KS, Zwingenberger AL, Theon AP, et al. Long-term survival with stereotactic radiotherapy for imaging-diagnosed pituitary tumors in dogs. Vet Radiol Ultrasound 2019;60:219–32. https://doi.org/10.1111/vru.12708.

26. Sanders K, Kooistra HS, Galac S. Treating canine Cushing's syndrome: Current options and future prospects. Vet J 2018;241:42–51.

27. Golinelli S, de Marco V, Leal RO, et al. Comparison of methods to monitor dogs with hypercortisolism treated with trilostane. J Vet Intern Med 2021;35:2616–27. https://doi.org/10.1111/jvim.16269.

28. Wood FD, Pollard RE, Uerling MR, et al. Diagnostic imaging findings and endocrine test results in dogs with pituitary-dependent hyperadrenocorticism that did or did not have neurologic abnormalities: 157 cases (1989–2005). J Am Vet Med Assoc 2007;231(7):1081–5.

29. Teshima T, Hara Y, Takekoshi S, et al. Trilostane-induced inhibition of cortisol secretion results in reduced negative feedback at the hypothalamic–pituitary axis. Domest Anim Endocrinol 2009;36:32–44. https://doi.org/10.1016/j.domaniend.2008.10.002.

30. Owen TJ, Chen AV, Martin LG. Why, when, how and post-operative care of dogs undergoing transsphenoidal hypophysectomy for large sellar masses. J Vet Intern Med 2016;30:1939.

31. Fracassi F, Mandrioli L, Shehdula D, et al. Complete surgical removal of a very enlarged pituitary corticotroph adenoma in a dog. J Am Anim Hosp Assoc 2014;50:192–7.

32. Del Magno S, Fracassi F, Grinwis GC, et al. Sequential treatment of a large pituitary corticotroph neoplasm and associated neurologic signs in a dog. J Am Anim Hosp Assoc 2019;55(2). 5522-e602.

33. Long SN, Michieletto A, Anderson TJ, et al. Suspect pituitary apoplexy in a German shorthaired pointer. J Small Anim Pract 2003;44:497–502. https://doi.org/10.1111/j.1748-5827.2003.tb00110.x.

34. Polledo L, Grinwis GCM, Graham P, et al. Pathological findings in the pituitary glands of dogs and cats. Vet Pathol 2018;55(6):880–8. https://doi.org/10.1177/0300985818784162.

35. Reusch CE, Burkhardt WA, Meier VS, et al. Acromegaly due to a pituitary tumor in a dog – diagnosis, therapy and long-term follow-up. Zurich Open Repository and Archive 2019. Schweizer Archiv für Tierheilkunde 2019;161(5):319–27.

36. Steele MMW, Lawson JS, Scudder C, et al. transsphenoidal hypophysectomy for the treatment of hypersomatotropism secondary to a pituitary somatotroph adenoma in a dog. J Vet Intern Med 2024;38:351–7.

37. Cosio C, Sartori E, Garatti M, et al. Prolactinoma in a dog. Vet Pathol 2017;54(6):972–6.

38. Van Rijn SJ, Galac S, Tryfonidou MA, et al. The influence of pituitary size on outcome after transsphenoidal hypophysectomy in a large cohort of dogs with pituitary-dependent hypercortisolism. J Vet Intern Med 2016;30:989–95.

39. Castillo VA, Pessina PP, Garcia JD, et al. Ectopic ACTH syndrome in a dog with a mesenteric neuroendocrine tumour: a case report. Vet Med 2014;59:352–8.

40. Galac S, Kooistra HS, Voorhout G, et al. Hyperadrenocorticism in a dog due to ectopic secretion of adrenocorticotropic hormone. Domest Anim Endocrinol 2005;28:338–48.
41. Churcher RK. Hepatic carcinoid, hypercortisolism and hypokalaemia in a dog. Aust Vet J 1999;77:641–5.
42. Fenn J, Kenny PJ, Scudder CJ, et al. Efficacy of hypophysectomy for the treatment of hypersomatotropism-induced diabetes mellitus in 68 cats. J Vet Intern Med 2021;35:823–33.
43. Van Bokhorst LK, Galac S, Kooistra HS, et al. Evaluation of hypophysectomy for treatment of hypersomatotropism in 25 cats. J Vet Intern Med 2021;35:834–42.
44. Meij BP, Van der Vlught-Meijer RH, Van den Ingh TSGAM, et al. Melanotroph pituitary adenoma in a cat with diabetes mellitus. Vet Pathol 2005;42:92–7.
45. Meij BP, Van der Vlught-Meijer RH, Van den Ingh TSGAM, et al. Somatotroph and corticotroph pituitary adenoma (double adenoma) in a cat with diabetes mellitus and hyperadrenocorticism. J comp Path 2004;130:209–15. https://doi.org/10.1016/j.jcpa.2003.09.004.
46. Teshima T, Hara Y, Shigihara K, et al. Coexistence of corticotroph adenoma and thyrotroph hyperplasia in a dog. J Vet Med Sci 2009;71(1):93–8.
47. Chae Y, Yun T, Koo Y, et al. Case report: Central-pituitary hypothyroidism concurrent with hyperadrenocorticism without pituitary macroadenoma in a Miniature Schnauzer dog. Front Vet Sci 2023;10:1257624. https://doi.org/10.3389/fvets.2023.1257624.
48. Owen TJ, Martin LG, Chen AV. Transsphenoidal surgery for pituitary tumors and other sellar masses. Vet Clin Small Anim 2018;48:129–51.
49. Van Bokhorst KL, Kooistra HS, Boroffka SAEB, et al. Concurrent pituitary and adrenocortical lesion son computed tomography imaging in dogs with spontaneous hypercortisolism. J Vet Inten Med 2019;33:72–8.
50. Van der Vlugt-Meijer RH, Meij BP, van den Ingh TS, et al. Dynamic computed tomography of the pituitary gland in dogs with pituitary-dependent hyperadrenocorticism. J Vet Intern Med 2003;17:773–80.
51. Sato A, Teshima T, Ishino H, et al. A magnetic resonance imaging-based classification system for indication if trans-sphenoidal hypophysectomy in canine pituitary-dependent hypercortisolism. J Small Anim Pract 2016;57:240–6.
52. Van Stee LL, van Rijn SJ, Galac S, et al. Challenges of transsphenoidal pituitary surgery in severe brachycephalic dogs. Front Vet Sci 2023;10:1154617. https://doi.org/10.3389/fvets.2023.1154617.
53. Florkow MC, Willemsen K, Zijlstra F, et al. MRI-based synthetic CT shows equivalence to conventional Ct for the morphological assessment of the hip joint. J Orthop Res 2022;40:954–64. https://doi.org/10.1002/jor.25127.
54. Paul R, Johansson R, Kiuru A, et al. Imaging of canine cancers with 18F-2-fluoro-2-deoxy-D-glucose (FDG) suggests further applications for cancer imaging in man. Nucl Med Commun 1984;5:641–6.
55. Hansen AE, McEvoy F, Engelholm SA, et al. FDG PET/CT imaging in canine cancer patients. Vet Radiol Ultrasound 2010;52(2):201–6.
56. Mondal SB, Cm O'Brien, Bishop K, et al. Repurposing molecular imaging and sensing for cancer image-guided surgery. J Nucl Med 2020;61:1113–22. https://doi.org/10.2967/jnumed.118.220426.
57. Yun T, Koo Y, Kim S, et al. Characteristics of 18F-FDG and 18F-FDOPA PET in an 8-year-old neutered male Yorkshire Terrier dog with glioma: long-term chemotherapy using hydroxyurea plus imatinib with prednisolone and immunoreactivity for PDGFR-β and LAT1. Vet Q 2021;41(1):163–71. https://doi.org/10.1080/01652176.2021.1906466.

58. Son Y, Kim D, Kang J, et al. CASE REPORT Open Access High-resolution fluoro-deoxyglucose positron emission tomography and magnetic resonance imaging findings of a pituitary microtumor in a dog. Ir Vet J 2015;68:22.
59. Macfarlane J, Bashari WQ, Senanayake R, et al. Advances in the imaging of pituitary tumors. Endocrinol Metab Clin N Am 2020;49:357–73.
60. Meij BP. Hypophysectomy as a treatment for canine and feline Cushing's disease. Vet Clin N Am 2001;31(5):1015–41.
61. Kooistra HS, Voorhout G, Mol JA, et al. Correlation between impairment of glucocorticoid feedback and the size of the pituitary gland in dogs with pituitary-dependent hyperadrenocorticism. J Endocrinol 1997;152:387–94.
62. Morsink NC, Klaassen NJM, Meij BP, et al. Case Report: Radioactive Holmium-166 Microspheres for the Intratumoral Treatment of a Canine Pituitary Tumor. Front Vet Sci 2021;8:748247. https://doi.org/10.3389/fvets.2021.748247.
63. Meij BP, Voorhout G, Van den Ingh TS, et al. Transsphenoidal hypophysectomy in beagle dogs: evaluation of a microsurgical technique. Vet Surg 1997;26:295–309.
64. Meij BP, Voorhout G, van den Ingh TSGAM, et al. Transsphenoidal hypophysectomy for treatment of pituitary-dependent hyperadrenocorticism in 7 cats. Vet Surg 2001;30:72–86.
65. Mamelak AN, Owen TJ, Bruyette D. Transsphenoidal surgery using a high definition video endoscope for pituitary adenomas in dogs with pituitary dependent hypercortisolism: methods and results. Vet Surg 2014;43:369–77.
66. Schmale IL, Vandelaar J, Luong AU, et al. Image-guided surgery and intraoperative imaging in rhinology: clinical update and current state of the art. Ear Nose Throat J 2021;100(10):NP475–86. https://doi.org/10.1177/0145561320928202.
67. Owen TJ, Chen AV, Frey S, et al. Transsphenoidal surgery; accuracy of an image-guided neuronavigation system to approach the pituitary fossa (sella turcica). Vet Surg 2018;47:664–71.
68. Roh Y, Kim D, Jeong S, et al. Evaluation of the accuracy of three-dimensionally printed patient-specific guides for transsphenoidal hypophysectomy in small-breed dogs. Am J Vet Res 2022;83:5.
69. Escauriaza L, Fenn J, McCue J, et al. A 3-dimensional printed patient specific surgical guide to facilitate transsphenoidal hypophysectomy in dogs. Front Vet Sci 2022;9:930856. https://doi.org/10.3389/fvets.2022.930856.
70. Micko A, Agam MS, Brunswick A, et al. Treatment strategies for giant pituitary adenomas in the era of endoscopic transsphenoidal surgery: a multicenter series. J Neurosurg 2022;136:776–85.
71. Tang OY, Hsueh WD, Anderson Eloy J, et al. Giant Pituitary Adenoma – Special Considerations. Otolaryngol Clin N Am 2022;55:351–79.
72. Makarenko S, Alzahrani I, Karsy M, et al. Outcomes and surgical nuances in management of giant pituitary adenomas: a review of 108 cases in the endoscopic era. J Neurosurg 2022;137:635–46.
73. Senior BA, Ebert CS, Bednarski KK, et al. Minimally invasive pituitary surgery. Laryngoscope 2008;118:1842–55. https://doi.org/10.1097/MLG.0b013e31817e2c43.
74. Hanson JM, Teske E, Voorhout G, et al. Prognostic factors for outcome after transsphenoidal hypophysectomy in dogs with pituitary-dependent hyperadernocortisolism. J Neurosurg 2007;107:830–40.
75. Hara Y. Transsphenoidal surgery in canines: safety, efficacy and patient selection. Vet Med Res Rep 2020;11:1–14. https://doi.org/10.2147/VMRR.S175995.
76. Lehner L, Czeibert K, Csöndes J, et al. Endoscope-guided transsphenoidal removal of a hypophyseal tumour in a dog. Case study. Magyar Állatorvosok Lapja 2018;140(9):535–50.

77. Rivenburg R, Owen TJ, Martin LG, et al. Pituitary surgery : changing the paradigm in veterinary medicine in the United States. J Am Anim Hosp Assoc 2021;57:73–80. https://doi.org/10.5326/JAAHA-MS-7009.

78. Staartjes VE, Togni-Pogliorini A, Stumpo V, et al. Impact of intraoperative magnetic resonance imaging on gross total resection, extent of resection, and residual tumor volume in pituitary surgery: systematic review and meta-analysis. Pituitary 2021;24(4):644–56.

79. Owens EA, Hyun H, Dost TL, et al. Near-Infrared Illumination of Native Tissues for Image-Guided Surgery. J Med Chem 2016;59:5311–23. https://doi.org/10.1021/acs.jmedchem.6b00038.

80. Litvak ZN, Zada G, Laws ER. Indocyanine green fluorescence endoscopy for visual differentiation of pituitary tumor from surrounding structures. J Neurosurg 2012;116:935–41.

81. Vergeer RA, Theunissen REP, van Elk T, et al. Fluorescence-guided detection of pituitary neuroendocrine tumor (PitNET) tissue during endoscopic transsphenoidal surgery available agents, their potential, and technical aspects. Rev Endocr Metab Disord 2022;23:647–57.

82. Aghapour M, Bockstahler B. State of the art and future prospectives of virtual and augmented reality in veterinary medicine: a systematic review. Animal 2022;12:3517.

83. Hunt JA, Heydenburg M, Anderson SL, et al. Does virtual reality training improve veterinary students' first canine surgical performance? Vet Rec 2020;186(17):562. https://doi.org/10.1136/vr.105749.

84. Zhou C, Zhu M, Shi Y, et al. Robot-assisted surgery for mandibular angle split osteotomy using augmented reality: preliminary results on clinical animal experiment. Aesthetic Plast Surg 2017;41:1228–36. https://doi.org/10.1007/s00266-017-0900-5.

85. Li C, Zheng Y, yuan Y, et al. Augmented reality navigation-guided pulmonary nodule localization in a canine model. Transl Lung Cancer Res 2021;10(11):4152–60. https://doi.org/10.21037/tlcr-21-618.

86. Ioannou I, Kazmierczak E, Stern L. Comparison of oral surgery task performance in a virtual reality surgical simulator and an animal model using objective measures. In 2015 37th Annual International Conference of the IEEE Engineering in Medicine and Biology Society (EMBC) 2015 Aug 25 (pp. 5114-5117). IEEE.

87. Wilkie N, McSorley G, Creighton C, et al. Mixed reality for veterinary medicine: Case study of a canine femoral nerve block. In: Medicine & Biology Society (EMBC)20. Montreal, QC, Canada: IEEE; 2020 Jul. p. 6074–7.

88. Shimada M, Kurihara K, Tsujii T. Prototype of an Augmented Reality System to Support Animal Surgery using HoloLens 2, 7. Japan: IEEE; Osaka; 2022 Mar. p. 335–7.

89. Baskaran V, Strkalj G, Strkalj M, et al. Current applications and future perspectives of the use of 3D printing in anatomical training and neurosurgery. Front Neuroanat 2016;10:69. https://doi.org/10.3389/fnana.2016.00069.

90. Vakharia VN, Vakharia NN, Hill CS. Review of 3-dimensional printing on cranial neurosurgery simulation training. World Neursurg 2016;88:188–98.

91. Riutort KT, Clifton W, Damon A, et al. Construction of an affordable lumbar neuraxial block model using 3d printed materials. Cureus 2019;11(10):e6033. https://doi.org/10.7759/cureus.6033.

92. Pearce P, Novak J, Wijesekera A, et al. Properties and implementation of 3-dimensionally printed models in spine surgery: a mixed-methods review with meta-analysis. World Neurosurg 2023;169:57–72.

93. Iqbal JM, Javed Z, Sadia H, et al. Clinical applications of artificial intelligence and machine learning in cancer diagnosis: looking into the future. Cancer Cell Int 2021;21:270.

94. Jones OT, Matin RN, van der Schaar M, et al. Artificial intelligence and machine learning algorithms for early detection of skin cancer in community and primary care settings: a systematic review. Lancet Digit Health 2022;4:e466–76.

95. Mendes J, Domingues J, Aidos H, et al. AI in breast cancer imaging: a survey of different applications. J Imaging 2022;8:228.

96. Lui J, Lei J, Ou Y, et al. Mammography diagnosis of breast cancer screening through machine learning: a systematic review and meta-analysis. Clin Exp Med 2023;23:2341–56.

Updates on Radiation Therapy for Pituitary Tumors
Techniques and Prognosis

Michael S. Kent, DVM, MAS, ECVDI (RO)[a],[*],[1], Matthias Rosseel, DVM[b],[1]

KEYWORDS

- Canine • Dog • Feline • Cat • Pituitary tumor • Radiation therapy

KEY POINTS

- Both dogs and cats with pituitary tumors can have an excellent response to treatment with radiation therapy.
- Dogs with current planning and protocols have better outcomes with conventionally fractionated radiation therapy as compared to stereotactic protocols.
- MRI may be better at delineating the tumor than contrast computed tomography scans.
- In general, radiation therapy for pituitary tumors has a very manageable side effect profile.

INTRODUCTION

The pituitary gland sits adjacent to the brain in the sella turcica, which is also called the pituitary fossa, which is a depression in the basisphenoid bone. Pituitary tumors are classified as either benign or malignant, with benign adenomas being much more common than malignant carcinomas.[1] Benign tumors can further be classified into adenomas and invasive adenomas.[2] Tumors can be either a microtumor or a macrotumor. While there is not a standardized method determining which tumors are classified as which, most people currently classify a pituitary tumor that extends dorsally above the sella turcica as being a macrotumor.[3]

CLINICAL PRESENTATION

Clinical signs related to pituitary tumors in dogs and cats are heavily dependent on the size and functional status of the tumor. Nonfunctional tumors often are identified as an underlying cause of progressive neurologic signs, including seizures, behavior

[a] Department of Surgical and Radiological Sciences, School of Veterinary Medicine, University of California Davis, Davis, CA, USA; [b] William R. Pritchard Veterinary Medical Teaching Hospital, School of Veterinary Medicine, University of California Davis, Davis, CA, USA
[1] Authors contributed equally to this work.
* Corresponding author.
E-mail address: mskent@ucdavis.edu

Vet Clin Small Anim 55 (2025) 119–133
https://doi.org/10.1016/j.cvsm.2024.07.010   **vetsmall.theclinics.com**

changes, blindness, circling, head pressing, and lethargy. These nonfunctional tumors often present as macrotumors. Functional tumors can present as either macrotumors or microtumors. In the case where a functional tumor is a macrotumor, it still has the potential to cause neurologic signs, and patients often present with endocrine abnormalities, namely pituitary-dependent hyperadrenocorticism (PDH) in dogs from a corticotroph adenoma and hypersomatotropism with secondary acromegaly in cats.[1] Other, less common, endocrine abnormalities have also been reported at the time of diagnosis. Pituitary tumors can also be found incidentally when performing advanced imaging on patients as part of a workup for a separate illness.

CURRENT EVIDENCE

Studies on using radiation therapy for the treatment of pituitary masses began with a canine case report presented in 1985.[4] Since then, imaging, treatment delivery methods, and radiation treatment planning modalities have progressed rapidly. Turn of the century treatment planning and delivery for pituitary tumors was limited via the technology available and was often delivered via equally weighted parallel-opposed fields. In time, this progressed from 4 field box treatments to 3 dimensional conformal radiotherapy and conformal arc therapy to intensity modulated radiation therapy (IMRT) to the latest technology focused on stereotactic radiation therapy (SRT) and stereotactic radiosurgery (SRS). The more advanced techniques allow for better targeting of the tumor and sparing of normal surrounding tissues. Examples of different treatment plan types for a canine pituitary tumor are shown in **Figs. 1** and **2**.

Canine

Goossens and colleagues[5] described a case series of 6 dogs with PDH treated with 4 Gy per fraction for 11 fraction therapy using a cobalt-60 machine. Tumor volumes were based off MR images and margins of 1 to 1.5 cm were used during treatment planning to ensure adequate tumor coverage. While only a single patient had a durable remission of clinical signs, the mass effect as measured by repeat MRI was significantly reduced in all patients 1 year out from treatment, indicating potential efficacy for nonfunctional tumors.

Théon and Feldman,[6] from the same group, evaluated the use of cobalt-60 megavoltage radiation at a similar time for the treatment of pituitary tumors specifically

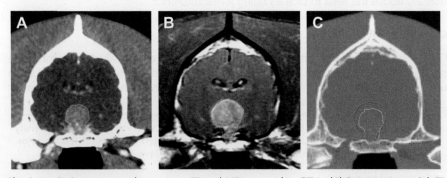

Fig. 1. A pituitary macroadenoma on CT and MRI vs overlap GTVs. (*A*) Postcontrast axial CT of a pituitary tumor contoured in blue. (*B*) T1 postcontrast axial MRI sequence with a pituitary tumor contoured in pink. (*C*) Noncontrast axial CT of the same patient showing GTV variation between blue (CT) and pink (MRI) showing an increase in the tumor size when visualize on MRI. CT, computed tomography; GTV, gross tumor volume.

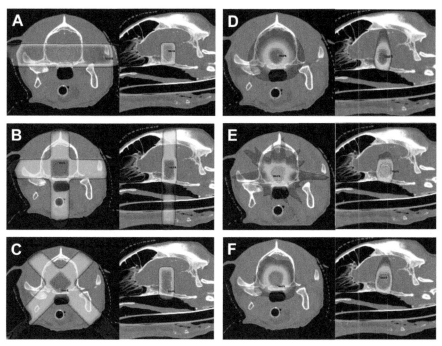

Fig. 2. Treatment plans for a canine pituitary tumor. Axial and sagittal noncontrast CT images depicting dose-color wash distribution using different computerized treatment planning techniques. Red areas indicate regions of higher dose while blue indicates low-dose areas. It can be seen that the more advanced treatment planning techniques provide more conformal coverage of the tumor and decreased dose to normal tissues such as the surrounding brain. (A) Parallel opposed; (B) 4 field box; (C) 4 field box diagonal; (D) conformal arc therapy; (E) 7 field IMRT; and (F) VMAT. The dose-color wash represents a gradient from 30% (blue) to >100% (red) of prescribed dose. CT, computed tomography; IMRT, intensity-modulated radiation therapy; VMAT, volumetric modulated arc therapy.

causing neurologic deficits. Their aims were to deliver 4 Gy per fraction for 12 fractions delivered 3 times weekly via parallel opposed fields in a larger population of 24 dogs. Ten of the 24 patients had complete resolution of neurologic signs with a median time to improvement of 16 days after starting treatment. Three patients, however, died during treatment from progressive neurologic disease and 1 additional dog died 23 days after completing therapy due to a similar cause.

Bley and colleagues[7] treated 46 dogs with brain tumors, 13 of which had an imaging-based diagnosis of a pituitary tumor, with a range of fractionations (10–17) and treatment modalities to reach a total dose of 35 to 45 Gy. Patients were treated with electrons, photons, or protons. Pituitary-specific data were not delineated; however, the greater population showed 95% of patients having some degree of improvement in neurologic signs. Tumor-specific survival data showed a median survival time (MST) of 1308 days for patients whose death could be attributed to their pituitary tumor and an MST of 688 days for all patients with pituitary tumors regardless of cause of death. No prognostic factors were significantly associated with survival for dogs with pituitary tumors in this patient population.

With the advent of safer anesthetic agents allowing for daily treatment of patients, Kent and colleagues[8] evaluated the use of daily fractionation in 19 dogs and paired these data with a control group of 27 dogs who received medical management only. Dogs were treated with parallel opposed fields; however, the addition of daily mega-voltage port films for positioning allowed for 1 cm margins. Treatment consisted of 16 daily fractions of 3 Gy for a total dose of 48 Gy using 4 MV photons. MST for dogs treated with this protocol was not reached with a mean survival time of 1405 days. MST in the medically managed group was significantly decreased at 359 days. Of the 14 dogs with PDH, 5 showed resolution of clinical signs as reported by the owners. Of the 14 patients with neurologic disease who completed treatment, 5 had complete resolution and 4 had transient resolution of signs. Two pieces of prognostic information came from this data set: maximum tumor to brain height ratio greater than 25% and tumor volume to brain volume ratio greater than 5% being negatively correlated with prognosis.

Mariani and colleagues[9] in 2015 provided the first information on SRS for pituitary tumors. Among their 51 dogs in the study with intracranial masses, 4 had pituitary tumors, and specific MST for these patients treated with a single fraction of 15 to 25 Gy was 118 days. The small population prevented further disease-specific analysis from being performed.

The first published description of a 4 field box technique for pituitary tumors was by Sawada and colleagues[10] in 2018 for 9 dogs with PDH. Advances in on-board imaging and treatment delivery accuracy allowed the reduction of treatment margins to 0.5 cm from the gross tumor volume (GTV) as delineated on MRI. Treatment protocols consisted of 4 Gy per fraction for 12 fractions on a Monday-Wednesday-Friday schedule. All 8 patients with neurologic signs prior to treatment saw either a complete resolution (4 patients) or a transient resolution (4 patients) of these signs. On repeat posttreatment MRI examination, half of the treated patients showed signs of pituitary hemorrhage. No significant difference was seen in circulating adrenocorticotropic hormone (ACTH) levels after treatment.

The use of SRT and SRS has been described in 2 publications focused on the treatment of canine pituitary tumors. Gieger and Nolan[11] described the use of a 16 Gy, single-fraction SRS technique in 13 dogs. Of these 13 patients, 9 showed improvement in neurologic deficits. Forty-six percent of the patients were still alive during data collection; however, the reported median overall survival time was 357 days. This is also the only publication that discusses contouring variations between postcontrast CT and MRI for pituitary tumors. MRI contour volumes were significantly larger, indicating that a clinical target volume (CTV) may be necessary if GTV contours are based solely on a postcontrast CT. A publication from Hansen and colleagues[12] had similar survival times with SRS and SRT protocols with a median overall survival time for 32 patients treated with a single fraction of 15 Gy and 12 patients treated with 3 fractions of 8 Gy being 311 days. No significant difference between the 2 protocols was found. For the 33 patient with neurologic signs pretreatment, 27 had improvement of these signs during the follow-up period.

The summarized literature surrounding radiation therapy for the treatment of canine pituitary tumors has been compiled in **Table 1**.

Feline

The treatment of feline pituitary tumors with radiation therapy was first published in 1990 by Peterson and colleagues.[13] They documented only 1 of 2 patients showing any improvement in neurologic signs or diabetes control with a similar protocol previously used in dogs. In 2002, Kaser-Hotz and colleagues[14] published a case series of 5 cats presenting with a mixture of neurologic signs and presumptive acromegaly. These cases were treated with electrons alone or electrons and photons in 3.5 to 4.0 Gy

Table 1
Published studies on the treatment of canine pituitary tumors with radiation therapy

Study, Study Type (Year Published)	Patient Number	Source and Dose/Protocol of Radiation	Outcomes
Goossens et al,[5] 1998. Retrospective case series	6	Cobalt-60; 44 Gy in 11 4 Gy fractions on a Monday-Wednesday-Friday schedule	PDH improved in 5 out of 6 patients (2 out of 6 had permanent CR, 1 transient CR). ACTH levels decreased in all 6. At 1 y, tumor size was down 25% in 2 out of 6 and not detectable in 4 out of 6
Théon et al,[6] 1998. Prospective clinical trial	24	Cobalt-60; 48 Gy in 12 4 Gy fractions on a Monday-Wednesday-Friday schedule	Neurologic clinical signs (CS): CR 10, PR 10, 4 died during or early after RT. PDH CS: 2 y control rate of PDH of 32%. Median control duration of 27.6 mo
Bley et al,[7] 2005. Retrospective case series	46 (13 pituitary)	Betatron 12–31 MeV electrons (12), 16 MeV electrons (31), 6 MV Dynaray LA20 (31), 138–160 MeV protons + electrons (2). Protons alone (1); 35–45 Gy total dose in 10–17 fractions on either a Monday-Wednesday-Friday or Monday-Tuesday-Thursday-Friday schedule; Proton delivery was 52.5 Gy in 15 fractions on a Monday-Tuesday-Thursday-Friday schedule	85% (33 out of 39) had improvement in neurologic signs within 3 wk of treatment (tx). 4 out of 39 (10%) reported improvement within 3 mo. Overall improvement in 95% of patients
Kent et al,[8] 2007. Retrospective case–control study	46	4 MV linear accelerator; 48 Gy in 16 3 Gy fractions on a Monday-Friday schedule	PDH: 6 out of 14 (40%) endocrine improvement; Neurologic: 14 with CS, 5 CR (35%), 4 transient resolution, 3 no change. Survival-treated: MST not reached. Mean ST 1,405 d; 1 y ST 93%, 2 y 87%, and 3 y 55%; Nontreated: MST 358 d. Mean ST 551 d; 1 y ST 45%, 2 y 32%, and 3 y 25%
de Fornel et al,[22] 2007. Retrospective case series	12	Cobalt-60 (n = 5) and 5 MV linear accelerator (n = 7); 36 Gy in 12 3 Gy fractions on either a Monday-Wednesday-Friday schedule (n = 8) or Tuesday-Thursday schedule (n = 4)	10 out of 11 dogs had >30% decrease in tumor height. 11 out of 11 dogs showed neurologic improvement. MST: 17.7 mo, Mean ST: 22.6 mo

(continued on next page)

Table 1
(continued)

Study, Study Type (Year Published)	Patient Number	Source and Dose/Protocol of Radiation	Outcomes
Mariani et al,[9] 2015. Retrospective case series	51 (4 pituitary)	6 MV linear accelerator; 15–25 Gy (median 16.25 Gy) in a single fraction	MST: 118 d (pituitary only) 1 y ST 0%
Marcinowska et al,[20] 2015. Prospective nonrandomized clinical trial	24	6 MV linear accelerator; 38 Gy in ten 3.8 Gy fractions on a Monday-Wednesday-Friday schedule (n = 12); or 38 Gy in a single 5 Gy dose followed by four 8.25 Gy fractions delivered once weekly (n = 12)	Group 1 (10 tx): 11 out of 12 clinical improvement; Group 2 (5 tx): 9 out of 12 clinical improvement; MST: 235 d
Savada et al,[10] 2018. Study type not described	9	4 MV linear accelerator; 48 Gy in twelve 4 Gy fractions on a Monday-Wednesday-Friday schedule	8 out of 9 showed neurologic improvement (4 CR); Significant decrease in pituitary:brain height; No change in basal ACTH; and MST: not published
Hansen et al,[12] 2019. Retrospective case series	45	6 MV linear accelerator; 15 Gy in a single fraction (n = 32); 24 Gy in 3 8 Gy fractions on consecutive day (n = 12); 24 Gy in three 8 Gy fractions on a Monday-Wednesday-Friday schedule (n = 1)	37 out of 45 clinical improvement; 9 out of 21 (reported) saw improvement in Cushing's signs/management; 27 out of 33 saw neurologic improvement; MST: 311 d
Gieger and Nolan,[11] 2021, Retrospective case series	13	6 MV linear accelerator; 16 Gy in a single fraction	9 out of 13 neurologic improvement; MST: 357 d 1 y ST 46%, 1.5 y 15%
Rapastella et al,[21] 2023. Multicenter retrospective cohort study	94	6 MV linear accelerator (36). Information not fully described (58); A median of 45 Gy (12–50) delivered in 3–20 fractions on a Monday-to-Friday or a Monday-Wednesday-Friday schedule (n = 80); A median of 37 Gy (29–48) delivered in 5 prescribed fractions (1–5 delivered) on a once weekly schedule (n = 14)	PDH: CS improved in 21 out of 37 patients MST: 514 d

Abbreviations: CR, complete response; CS, clinical signs; Gy, Gray; MeV, megaelectron volt; MST, median survival time; MV, megavolt; PDH, pituitary-dependent hyperadrenocorticism; PR, partial response; ST, survival time.

fractions on a Monday, Wednesday, Friday basis for a total of 10 to 12 fractions. The limited numbers in this case series limited robust statistical analysis, but all 5 patients saw clinical benefit. Further, a tumor volume reduction or stable disease was seen in the 4 cats that had follow-up CT scans. Survival times ranged from 5.5 to 20.5 months.

In 2006, Brearley and colleagues[15] reported 12 cats with a mixture of neurologic signs and uncontrolled diabetes mellitus that had undergone once weekly radiation therapy. Six of the 8 patients on insulin therapy saw a lifelong, durable reduction in insulin requirements with 5 being able to stop insulin therapy altogether. The remaining 2 patients saw a stabilization in insulin dosing. Around the same time, Mayer and colleagues[16] evaluated the use of conventionally fractionated radiation therapy over 15 to 19 treatments. Patient overall survival times were similar to those previously reported at 523 days; however, the response of diabetes mellitus and insulin requirements were less effective with 5 out of the 6 patients with diabetes still requiring insulin therapy.

In 2008, Sellon and colleagues[17] described the first use of SRS for the treatment of feline pituitary tumors with a single 15 Gy fraction. Five out of the 9 patients with diabetes mellitus saw some degree of insulin requirement reduction with the other 4 seeing no response. The 2 patients evaluated with neurologic signs showed dramatic and durable improvement. These cats had a MST of 29.4 months.

More recently, Wormhoudt and colleagues[18] described 53 cats with pituitary tumors treated with SRT with most receiving 3 fractions of 8 Gy using a 7 field IMRT plan. This data set showed the strongest response with 39 out of 41 cats with follow-up data showing a reduction in insulin requirement and roughly a third of them attaining either a partial or complete remission. They reported that the median time to maximal response, defined as the lowest insulin requirement, was roughly 9.5 months. Additionally, they reported the longest MST for this disease at 1071 days. IGF-1 concentration, pituitary height, and age were evaluated for prognostic significance with only age being negatively correlated with survival time.

The summarized literature surrounding radiation therapy for the treatment of feline pituitary tumors has been compiled in **Table 2**.

ADVERSE EVENTS

Radiation therapy adverse events are traditionally temporally separated into 3 categories: acute, delayed acute, and late. **Table 3** lists all published potential adverse events associated with radiation therapy for pituitary tumors in both dogs and cats.

Acute radiation reactions occur during or within weeks of completing radiation therapy and are believed to be secondary to both intratumoral and peritumoral edema. This often presents as the development or worsening of pre-existing neurologic signs. Reported literature concerning acute radiation reaction in dogs is variable with some showing no acute reactions, and others describing up to a 22% incidence, with worsening neurologic signs being the most common. Other reported acute reactions include alopecia, tremors, acute onset blindness, hypernatremia, and death during the course of treatment. In cats, the reported incidence of acute radiation effects is below 20% with mental dullness, light sensitivity, mydriasis, and death being reported. Management is often corticosteroid based but can include additional medications, such as mannitol in more severe cases.

Delayed acute reactions span from weeks to several months after completion of treatment and present often as a transient worsening of neurologic deficits. Historic literature has attributed these clinical signs primarily to a transient demyelination. These reactions have not been published in dogs with radiation therapy for pituitary tumors. Delayed acute effects have been reported in 2 cats that had undergone treatment, with one

Table 2
Published studies on the treatment of feline pituitary tumors with radiation therapy

Study, Study Type (Year Published)	Patient Number	Source and Dose/Protocol of Radiation	Outcomes
Peterson et al,[13] 1990. Study type not described	14 (only 2 RT patients)	Cobalt-60; 48 Gy in twelve 4 Gy fractions on a Monday-Wednesday-Friday schedule	Patient 1: 50% reduction in tumor size with resolution of neurologic signs and 6 mo of improved insulin resistance Patient 2: no response
Kaser-Hotz et al,[14] 2002. Study type not described	5	31 MeV electrons (5), 6 MV linear accelerator (1); 10–12 fractions of 3.5–4 Gy (20–30 MeV, n = 4); 5 fractions of 3.5 Gy (30 MeV) followed by 6 fractions of 3.5 Gy (6 MV, n = 1)	All patients had some neurologic improvement. 2 out of 5 patients died from progressive disease/late reaction MST: not published
Brearley et al,[15] 2006. Retrospective case series	12	4 MV linear accelerator; 37 Gy in a single 5 Gy dose followed by four 8 Gy fractions delivered once weekly	1 patient died during therapy MST: 72.3 wk
Mayer et al,[16] 2006. Retrospective case series	8	6 MV linear accelerator; 45 Gy in fifteen 3 Gy fractions on a Monday-Friday schedule (n = 3); 18–20 fractions of 2.7–3.0 Gy on a Monday-Friday schedule (n = 4); 51.3 Gy in nineteen 2.7 Gy fractions on Monday-Friday schedule (n = 1)	Clinical signs for DM improved in all cats, but 5 out of 6 required insulin to some degree for remainder of their lives (remaining patient had a suspected insulinoma) MST: 523 d
Sellon et al,[17] 2009. Retrospective case series	11	6 MV linear accelerator (10) or 10 MV linear accelerator (n = 1); 15 Gy in a single fraction (n = 8); 30 Gy in 2 15 Gy fractions (6 wk and 3 mo apart, respectively) (n = 2); 50 Gy in a single 15 Gy fraction followed by a single 20 Gy fractions 8 wk later followed by a single 15 Gy fraction 40 mo thereafter (n = 1)	2 out of 11 transient insulin independence, 3 out of 11 decrease in insulin dose, 4 out of 11 no improvement 2 out of 2 improvement in neuro signs (vision and aggression 1 out of 1) MST: 29.4 mo
Wormhoudt et al,[18] 2018. Retrospective case series	53	6 MV linear accelerator; 28 Gy in 4 7 Gy fractions delivered over consecutive days (n = 7); 27 Gy in four 6.75 fractions delivered over consecutive days (n = 3); 24 Gy in three 8 Gy fractions over consecutive days (n = 44); 18 Gy in 3 6 Gy fractions over consecutive days (n = 1); 17 Gy in a single fraction (n = 1)	95% (39 out of 41) required less insulin w/ 13 out of 41 (32%) being in remission. Permanent remission in 8 out of 13 14% (7) of treated developed hypothyroidism MST: 1071 d

| Körner et al,[23] 2019. Retrospective, multicenter case series | 22 (8 pituitary) | 6 MV linear accelerator; 40 Gy in ten 4 Gy fractions on a Monday-Friday schedule (n = 1); 42 Gy in ten 4.2 Gy fractions on a Monday-Friday schedule (n = 2); 42 Gy in fourteen 3 Gy fractions on a Monday-Friday schedule (n = 3); 42.5 Gy in seventeen 2.5 Gy fractions on a Monday-Friday schedule (n = 1); 45 Gy in twenty 2.25 Gy fractions on a Monday-Friday schedule (n = 1) | 21 out of 22 cats showed clinical and neurologic status improvements PFS for all cases was 510 d 1 y and 2 y survival: 56%, 37% MST: 515 d |

Abbreviations: DM, diabetes mellitus; Gy, Gray; MST, median survival time; RT, radiation therapy.

Table 3
Reported adverse events associated with radiation therapy for pituitary tumors in dogs and cats

	Dogs	Cats
Acute	Epilation/alopecia Otitis Anisocoria Deterioration of neurologic signs Hypernatremia Tremors Blindness Labored breathing without pneumonia Cushing's reflex Death	Epilation Mental dullness Light sensitivity Mydriasis Death
Delayed acute	No data published	Dullness Ataxia Stiffness of limbs and tail Hypermetria Behavior change Pain/discomfort
Late	Leukotrichia Hearing loss (either partial or complete) Vision loss without cataracts Progressive neurologic signs Secondary tumor formation Progressive bilateral temporal amyotrophia Hypothyroidism Diabetes insipidus Otitis media	Cataracts Hearing loss (either partial or complete) Vision loss without cataracts Hypothyroidism Progressive neurologic signs

showing a transient worsening of neurologic signs including dullness, ataxia, stiffness of limbs and tail, and hypermetria that resolved after 2 weeks. The other patient was euthanized 4 weeks after completing SRS for behavior changes and signs of pain or discomfort. The addition of corticosteroids may assist in reducing the clinical signs.

Late radiation reactions occur at least 3 months after treatment and, while less common than other reactions, consist of more serious side effects affecting quality of life.[19] These reactions are often a consequence of necrosis of the normal brain parenchyma. Late radiation reactions can mimic the initial presenting neurologic signs and can be challenging or impossible to fully differentiate from tumor recurrence, even with advanced imaging. Late reactions published for dogs include leukotrichia, hypernatremia, blindness, otitis media, hemorrhage within the tumor as seen on MRI, and development of other endocrinopathies, namely hypothyroidism and central diabetes insipidus.[6,8,10,12,20,21] There is a single report of a dog developing a thalamic mass within the irradiated field 217 days after completing therapy, which was likely a radiation-induced tumor.[8] Late reactions have been uncommonly reported in cats, but include hypothyroidism, cataracts, vision loss without cataracts, change in hearing, and onset of neurologic signs. Management of late reactions is aimed at controlling clinical signs for their respective presentations.

DISCUSSION

Radiation therapy for the treatment of canine pituitary tumors has been well reported with varying degrees of efficacy. When defining efficacy as purely increasing survival times, conventionally fractionated radiation therapy appears to provide the greatest benefit with medical management alone potentially providing similar survival times to the patients treated with either SRS or SRT. However, this viewpoint fails to include the benefit of increased quality of life that can come from alleviating clinical signs, whether they be neurologic, endocrine, or both. Despite the lack of prolonged survival times, SRT and SRS appear to provide significant improvement in clinical signs with a single fraction of 16 Gy helping improve 9 out of 13 patients treated and either a single fraction of 15 Gy or 3 fractions of 8 Gy showing improvement in 37 out of 45 dogs. Regardless of protocol, improvement of neurologic or endocrine clinical signs, whether transient or durable, is highly variable among various publications. Time to improvement of clinical signs is also highly variable with documented responses occurring as early as during treatment courses or taking up to a year after treatment. This variation in response between conventionally fractionated and stereotactic protocols requires further investigation with a potential explanation being a geographic miss given the strict margins required by stereotactic treatment. Minimum field sizes for the earlier machines were usually 3×3 cm^2 or 4×4 cm^2 which, in small patients, can be a substantial proportion of the calvarium. This often provided large margins around tumors compared with SRS or SRT planning margins that generally will limit the margin below a 2 mm expansion from the GTV. This is further complicated by the differences in tumor volumes found on CT and MRI. Most studies used contrast CT scans to identify the target. Had MRI been used, the tumor volume treated would have been larger minimizing the potential for a geographic miss leading to an early treatment failure. Another consideration for the difference would be if canine pituitary tumors simply respond better to conventional fractionation. The alpha/beta ratio, a measurement of tissue sensitivity to a change in dose per fraction, has not been evaluated in canine pituitary tumors and could provide data in determining optimal fractionation protocols.

The treatment of feline pituitary tumors appears to present contradictory information to the canine population, which is not entirely surprising given the different tumor tissue origins for their respective functional tumors. The highest published MST in cats was with an SRT protocol at 1071 days, which also showed 95% of patients having a reduction in insulin requirement with only a handful entering a permanent remission. This improvement in endocrine control is echoed in the other recently published literature that utilized a more fractionated protocol; however, MSTs with these protocols are reported at 515 and 523 days, respectively. Unlike the SRT data set in cats, there has not been a single large population of cats evaluated for the efficacy of conventionally fractionated radiation therapy.

Prognostic information has been investigated in both dogs and, to a lesser extent, cats. The canine data that are prognostic for survival are mixed given the various institutions, patient populations, and protocols. There are a few markers that have shown significance on occasion. Increased severity of neurologic signs at the time of diagnosis was found by both Théon and colleagues and Marcinowska and colleagues[20] to be significantly associated with decreased survival. Additionally, Kent and colleagues[8] showed that pituitary-to-brain height ratio greater than 25% and pituitary-to-brain volume ratio greater than 5% were associated with worse survival in their cohort of patients treated with conventionally fractionated radiation therapy. The articles analyzing SRT and SRS were unable to show significance for pituitary-to-brain height ratio; however, Hansen and colleagues[12] found GTV and PTV to brain volume ratio to be negatively correlated with survival. Protocol types have been evaluated with Marcinowska and colleagues[20] showing significant improvement in survival for patients treated with a 10 fraction protocol compared to a 5 fraction protocol utilizing the same total dose. Additionally, Rapastella and colleagues[21] showed that their definitive intent protocols had better survival times than their palliative protocols. The evaluation of functional status and their impact on survival has also shown mixed results. Hansen and colleagues[12] found that patients with PDH had significantly shorter survival time than their counterparts, whereas Rapastella and colleagues[21] showed no statistical difference in survival. In cats, the only data point among all publications found to have a significant negative impact on survival times has been the age of the patient.[18] Wormhoudt and colleagues found this correlation in cats undergoing SRT, where they also investigated IGF-1 levels and pituitary volume but were unable to show significant negative correlation with survival time.

Adverse effects associated with radiation therapy in dogs appear to be minimal and well tolerated with acute effects being the most common and the most easily addressed with corticosteroid supplementation. Delayed acute effects have not been published. Late effects, as mentioned previously, are challenging if not impossible to differentiate from tumor recurrence leading to a high incidence of deterioration of neurologic signs listed as potential late effects. Reported rates of treatment reactions in cats are similarly uncommon with acute reactions being the most widely reported in up to 18% of patients.[18] Acute delayed and late effects have been rarely reported in the feline literature with neurologic deterioration and endocrine disease being the most common.

Older radiation therapy machines did not have onboard imaging and were further limited by larger minimal field sizes. While this limited the risk of geographic miss, large volumes of normal brain would be irradiated. With the development of technology allowing for submillimeter positioning accuracy and the advent of SRT and SRS planning and delivery techniques, it is critical to note the results of Gieger and Nolan's analysis of variation in GTV based on imaging modality. MRI showed a larger tumor volume and more accurate tumor margins when contouring. For institutions without access to an MRI, Geiger and Nolan recommend the use of a contrast CT-based CTV to account for the imaging differences and minimize the risk of a geographic miss.

RECOMMENDATIONS

Currently, the recommended course of action for pituitary tumors being treated with radiation therapy relies on multiple factors, including the patient, client, and veterinary hospital's capabilities. When guiding clients through the complexity of choosing a stereotactic versus a conventionally fractionated protocol, multiple considerations need to be made.

- Patient comorbidities
- Patient anesthetic risk
- Patient temperament and impact on quality of life when visiting the hospital daily
- Client goals for the patient
- Client's ability to transport the patient
- Client perceived impact on quality of life
- Cost of various protocols
- The hospital having appropriate equipment to deliver SRT or SRS
- Appropriate staffing for specific protocols

These are just a few considerations that should be entertained when deciding on an appropriate protocol. When possible, the authors recommend a finely fractionated definitive course of radiation therapy for canine patients given the better published outcomes for both functional and nonfunctional pituitary tumors. Conventionally fractionated radiation therapy also allows for greater margins to be placed around the GTV, reducing the risk of geographic miss while minimizing the risk of late effects. The authors also recommend both thin-slice MRI sequences and contrast CT to help guide contouring when available. If contours are being made based on contrast CT alone, the authors recommend the use of a CTV to limit the risk of geographic miss.

Very similar considerations apply for feline patients when deciding between protocols. However, there have yet to be any large studies evaluating the potential benefits of conventionally fractionated radiation therapy. The largest population evaluated currently is a cohort of 8 cats. Therefore, the authors continue to offer both conventionally fractionated radiation therapy and SRT. There is some evidence that cats undergoing conventionally fractionated therapy have a quicker response in terms of insulin reduction than with stereotactic protocols. For contouring purposes, despite no studies evaluating tumor volume variations between contrast CT and MRI, both are recommended. When CT alone is used, a similar CTV recommendation is made as is for canine patients.

For all patients with pituitary tumors, cotreatment with an anti-inflammatory dose of corticosteroids through the course of treatment is recommended. With conventionally fractionated protocols in dogs without neurologic signs corticosteroid treatment is often delayed until midway through the course of treatment unlike with stereotactic protocols where treatment is generally begun prior to treatment. Tapering corticosteroids can begin as early as 2 to 4 weeks after completion of treatment if the patient is neurologically stable and is able to tolerate it. A slow taper over the course of an additional 2 to 4 weeks allows time to ensure that patients are tolerating the taper appropriately. Corticosteroid administration and its tapering must always be weighed against the patient's clinical picture, particularly in cats, where corticosteroids have been documented to lead to worsening heart disease and insulin resistance.

Monitoring after treatment is recommended to be aggressive shortly after completing treatment to evaluate for acute radiation reactions and allow for intervention when needed. The veterinarian who is managing the functional aspect of certain tumors should be informed that the treatment has been performed to limit the risk of overcorrection of the functional process and assist in monitoring for late radiation reaction. Repeat advanced imaging is at the discretion of the attending clinician, but is not recommended until 3 months after completing treatment and then every 3 to 6 months thereafter for clients who wish to be aggressive. For most patients, repeat imaging does not occur until the return of clinical signs during which it can be hard to evaluate changes in tumor characteristics since treatment.

SUMMARY

In summary, dogs and cats diagnosed with pituitary macrotumors are likely to benefit from radiation therapy. For dogs with tumors creating a mass effect and causing neurologic signs treatment with radiation therapy has the potential for a dramatic improvement in quality of life. For dogs with PDH, the literature is variable regarding response rates and duration with up to about a third of treatments having long-term endocrine control. For feline patients, radiation therapy appears to provide significant benefit with a potential increased benefit to the functional tumors that is not seen in dogs. Definitive intent fractionated protocols in dogs provide the longest survival times. The role of SRT remains open with alternative fractionation, and the use of increased margins is still being investigated. Side effect profiles in both dogs and cats appear minimal with corticosteroids helping reduce secondary edema in the short term.

CLINICS CARE POINTS

- While both SRT/SRS and conventionally fractionated radiation therapy have the ability to help control clinical signs in dogs with either functional or nonfunctional pituitary tumors, only conventionally fractionated radiation therapy has been shown to have a positive impact on MST. Tumor size is also prognostic, with those dogs having larger tumors more likely having shorter survivals.

- For cats, the most common presenting complaints relate to insulin-resistant diabetes mellitus although some tumors are nonfunctional. While survival and clinical response data are limited, particularly for conventionally fractionated radiation therapy protocols, it appears that cats may respond similarly between conventionally fractionated and SRS/SRT protocols. However, cats treated with conventionally fractionated protocols may have faster and perhaps more durable endocrine control.

- Concurrent treatment with an anti-inflammatory dose of corticosteroids, while not without risk, has a great potential to limit the deterioration of neurologic signs during the acute radiation reaction phase. This is particularly essential for those animals receiving stereotactic protocols.

- Contouring margins should be carefully considered when planning from a contrast CT alone without MRI, as CT is thought to underestimate true tumor volume.

DISCLOSURE

The authors have nothing to disclose.

REFERENCES

1. Sanders K, Galac S, Meij BP. Pituitary tumour types in dogs and cats. Vet J 2021; 270:105623. https://doi.org/10.1016/j.tvjl.2021.105623.
2. Pollard RE, Reilly CM, Uerling MR, et al. Cross-sectional imaging characteristics of pituitary adenomas, invasive adenomas and adenocarcinomas in dogs: 33 cases (1988-2006). J Vet Intern Med 2010;24(1):160–5. https://doi.org/10.1111/j.1939-1676.2009.0414.x.
3. Belka C, Budach W, Kortmann RD, et al. Radiation induced CNS toxicity–molecular and cellular mechanisms. Br J Cancer 2001;85(9):1233–9. https://doi.org/10.1054/bjoc.2001.2100.
4. FELDMAN EC, TURREL JM, NELSON RW. Radiation therapy of an ACTH-secreting pituitary hypothalamic mass - a case report. American College of Veterinary Internal Medicine 3rd annual forum 1985;140. San Diego.
5. Goossens MM, Feldman EC, Theon AP, et al. Efficacy of cobalt 60 radiotherapy in dogs with pituitary-dependent hyperadrenocorticism. J Am Vet Med Assoc 1998; 212(3):374–6.
6. Theon AP, Feldman EC. Megavoltage irradiation of pituitary macrotumors in dogs with neurologic signs. J Am Vet Med Assoc 1998;213(2):225–31.
7. Bley CR, Sumova A, Roos M, et al. Irradiation of brain tumors in dogs with neurologic disease. J Vet Intern Med 2005;19(6):849–54. https://doi.org/10.1892/0891-6640(2005)19[849:iobtid]2.0.co;2.
8. Kent MS, Bommarito D, Feldman E, et al. Survival, neurologic response, and prognostic factors in dogs with pituitary masses treated with radiation therapy and untreated dogs. J Vet Intern Med 2007;21(5):1027–33. https://doi.org/10.1892/0891-6640(2007)21[1027:snrapf]2.0.co;2.

9. Mariani CL, Schubert TA, House RA, et al. Frameless stereotactic radiosurgery for the treatment of primary intracranial tumours in dogs. Vet Comp Oncol 2015; 13(4):409–23. https://doi.org/10.1111/vco.12056.

10. Sawada H, Mori A, Lee P, et al. Pituitary size alteration and adverse effects of radiation therapy performed in 9 dogs with pituitary-dependent hypercortisolism. Res Vet Sci 2018;118:19–26. https://doi.org/10.1016/j.rvsc.2018.01.001.

11. Gieger TL, Nolan MW. Treatment outcomes and target delineation utilizing CT and MRI in 13 dogs treated with a uniform stereotactic radiation therapy protocol (16 Gy single fraction) for pituitary masses: (2014-2017). Vet Comp Oncol 2021;19(1):17–24. https://doi.org/10.1111/vco.12627.

12. Hansen KS, Zwingenberger AL, Theon AP, et al. Long-term survival with stereotactic radiotherapy for imaging-diagnosed pituitary tumors in dogs. Vet Radiol Ultrasound 2019;60(2):219–32. https://doi.org/10.1111/vru.12708.

13. Peterson ME, Taylor RS, Greco DS, et al. Acromegaly in 14 cats. J Vet Intern Med 1990;4(4):192–201. https://doi.org/10.1111/j.1939-1676.1990.tb00897.x.

14. Kaser-Hotz B, Rohrer CR, Stankeova S, et al. Radiotherapy of pituitary tumours in five cats. J Small Anim Pract 2002;43(7):303–7. https://doi.org/10.1111/j.1748-5827.2002.tb00078.x.

15. Brearley MJ, Polton GA, Littler RM, et al. Coarse fractionated radiation therapy for pituitary tumours in cats: a retrospective study of 12 cases. Vet Comp Oncol 2006;4(4):209–17. https://doi.org/10.1111/j.1476-5829.2006.00108.x.

16. Mayer MN, Greco DS, LaRue SM. Outcomes of pituitary tumor irradiation in cats. J Vet Intern Med 2006;20(5):1151–4. https://doi.org/10.1892/0891-6640(2006)20 [1151:ooptii]2.0.co;2.

17. Sellon RK, Fidel J, Houston R, et al. Linear-accelerator-based modified radiosurgical treatment of pituitary tumors in cats: 11 cases (1997-2008). J Vet Intern Med 2009;23(5):1038–44. https://doi.org/10.1111/j.1939-1676.2009.0350.x.

18. Wormhoudt TL, Boss MK, Lunn K, et al. Stereotactic radiation therapy for the treatment of functional pituitary adenomas associated with feline acromegaly. J Vet Intern Med 2018;32(4):1383–91. https://doi.org/10.1111/jvim.15212.

19. Poirier VJ, Keyerleber M, Gordon IK, et al. ACVR and ECVDI consensus statement: Reporting elements for toxicity criteria of the veterinary radiation therapy oncology group v2.0. Vet Radiol Ultrasound 2023;64(5):789–97. https://doi.org/10.1111/vru.13291.

20. Marcinowska A, Warland J, Brearley M, et al. Comparison of Two Coarse Fractionated Radiation Protocols for the Management of Canine Pituitary Macrotumor: An Observational Study of 24 Dogs. Vet Radiol Ultrasound 2015;56(5):554–62. https://doi.org/10.1111/vru.12270.

21. Rapastella S, Morabito S, Sharman M, et al. Effect of pituitary-dependent hypercortisolism on the survival of dogs treated with radiotherapy for pituitary macroadenomas. J Vet Intern Med 2023;37(4):1331–40. https://doi.org/10.1111/jvim.16724.

22. de Fornel P, Delisle F, Devauchelle P, Rosenberg D. Effects of radiotherapy on pituitary corticotroph macrotumors in dogs: a retrospective study of 12 cases. Can Vet J 2007;48(5):481–6.

23. Körner M, Roos M, Meier VS, et al. Radiation therapy for intracranial tumours in cats with neurological signs. J Feline Med Surg 2019;21(8):765–71.

Ventriculoperitoneal Shunting for Brain Tumors

Katharine Russell, MVB, Simon T. Kornberg, BVSc, DACVIM (Neurology)*

KEYWORDS

- Ventriculoperitoneal shunting • Brain tumors • Obstructive hydrocephalus

KEY POINTS

- VP shunting is considered the gold standard surgical intervention for managing obstructive hydrocephalus.
- VP shunting may improve quality of life and survival times in patients with obstructive hydrocephalus secondary to brain tumors.
- VP shunting can provide rapid, effective and durable relief from the clinical signs of obstructive hydrocephalus secondary to brain tumors when used alone, but is more effective alongside other treatment modalities.

INTRODUCTION

Brain tumors exert their clinical effects in a variety of ways. Mass effect, edema, seizures, and the vicious cycle of cause and effect are often the focus of therapeutic interventions employed to improve clinical signs and increase survival time. Obstructive hydrocephalus is a relatively common sequela of certain types of brain tumors and is often the major driver of clinical signs associated with tumors arising within the ventricular system. Due to the limited instances in which this syndrome is typically seen, the most effective treatment options are often not considered within our standard battery of therapeutic modalities for managing brain tumors.

Ventriculoperitoneal (VP) shunting is considered the gold standard surgical intervention for the management of obstructive hydrocephalus. It involves inserting a catheter through a small burr hole in the skull, which is then attached to a fixed or variable pressure valve. This valve then attaches to rubber tubing, which is passed subcutaneously and typically terminates within the abdomen. This apparatus facilitates drainage of the lateral and third ventricles to maintain an appropriate physiologic ventricular pressure. The technique can alleviate clinical signs associated with increased intraventricular pressure, as is seen in obstructive hydrocephalus. It is generally considered an effective and safe therapeutic intervention; however, there is a relatively high complication

Southeast Veterinary Neurology, 9300 Southwest 40th Street, Miami, FL 33165, USA
* Corresponding author.
E-mail address: DrKornberg@sevneurology.com

Vet Clin Small Anim 55 (2025) 135–147
https://doi.org/10.1016/j.cvsm.2024.07.011
0195-5616/25/© 2024 Elsevier Inc. All rights reserved, including those for text and data mining,
AI training, and similar technologies.

rate, which may require either removal or replacement of the shunt. Despite the complication rate, VP shunting can be used as an adjunctive treatment or emergency intervention alongside other treatments (eg, radiation, chemotherapy, or surgery) to provide rapid, effective, and durable relief from clinical signs of hydrocephalus in certain patients with brain tumors.

PATHOPHYSIOLOGY OF ACUTE OBSTRUCTIVE HYDROCEPHALUS

Acute obstructive hydrocephalus is a recognized potential sequela to intracranial neoplasms. Hydrocephalus may occur in the presence of intracranial tumors secondary to cerebrospinal fluid (CSF) outflow obstruction, poor CSF reabsorption, or increased CSF production.[1] Almost all instances of hydrocephalus are due to the obstruction of CSF flow with the rare exception being overproduction of CSF reported secondary to some choroid plexus tumors.[2] The rate that CSF is produced within the healthy brain is generally considered to be constant and will occur independent of intracranial pressure (ICP). In slowly progressing chronic hydrocephalus, there is time for the formation of alternative pathways for CSF absorption, which can help allow for normalization of ventricular pressure. With acute changes in CSF production or drainage, there is not enough time for these alternative pathways to form, so pressure within the ventricles rapidly rises resulting in clinical hydrocephalus. Brain damage is typically due to the effects of compressive and shear forces on the parenchyma, in addition to indirect injury caused by damage to the blood vessels. Over time this can lead to cortical destruction.[2] In more chronic cases, this will be seen as severe ventriculomegaly with a thin rim of cortical tissue and destruction of the septum pellucidum. This is not typical of acute hydrocephalus, such as those caused by neoplasia, as there has been little time for adaptation. This change in pressure within the ventricles can result in periventricular interstitial edema, which can be observed on cross-sectional imaging and can be used as a marker to help identify clinically significant ventriculomegaly and hypertensive hydrocephalus.[3]

Clinical hydrocephalus has been recognized with many tumor types but is most commonly associated with tumors of the ventricular system. In dogs, choroid plexus tumors make up approximately 10% of all primary intracranial tumors but only 0.6% of primary intracranial tumors in cats. Ventriculomegaly and hydrocephalus are seen in the majority of patients with choroid plexus tumors, and these are the most common causes of acute obstructive hydrocephalus secondary to neoplasia in the dog.[4,5] Ependymal tumors, while rare in dogs, are more common than choroid plexus tumors in cats, making up approximately 4% of feline primary intracranial tumors.[4,5] Meningiomas can occasionally arise from the tela choroidea within the ventricular system, particularly of the third ventricle where they have the potential to block CSF flow.[4] Tumors arising from the sella turcica can result in hydrocephalus if dorsal expansion is significant enough to compress the mesencephalic aqueduct. This has been associated with pituitary macroadenomas, meningiomas, lymphomas, germinomas, and craniopharyngiomas.[4] Rare instances of primitive neuroectodermal tumors expanding into the fourth ventricle have also been reported as a cause for obstructive hydrocephalus in animals.[4]

CASE SELECTION

Patients with brain tumors and progressive clinical signs occurring secondary to obstructive hydrocephalus are the target candidates for shunt placement. Typically, these patients will present localizing to the prosencephalon with signs such as seizures, blindness, behavior changes, and/or circling. Occasionally, these patients may present emergently with an acute and severe neurologic decline, necessitating urgent intervention. Patients with nonprogressive or stable clinical signs are typically not considered for treatment. In a small case series,[6] patients with obstructive hydrocephalus secondary to intraventricular tumors treated only palliatively with shunting had a similar median survival time as patients who received radiation therapy without VP shunt. This suggests that the application of a VP shunt has standalone efficacy in increasing survival and quality of life in these patients. However, median survival times in patients that had a VP shunt placed in addition to follow-up radiation therapy was significantly longer than median survival times in patients that had either radiation therapy or VP shunt alone. This suggests that the application of both therapeutic modalities is preferable to treat the underlying cause of the hydrocephalus whenever possible. This combination allows for treatment of the tumor in addition to acute relief of ICP. Timing of surgery is important for treatment success. Ideally, a shunt is placed in a clinical patient prior to undergoing radiation therapy or frequent anesthesia events in order to reduce anesthetic risk. In studies evaluating VP shunt placement prior to radiation therapy, patients were less likely to experience sudden death during the radiation procedure.[7] Radiation therapy, surgery, and chemotherapy should all be considered as part of a comprehensive treatment plan addressing the underlying cause of the clinical signs.

DIAGNOSTICS AND PREOPERATIVE PLANNING

There are several ways in which a diagnosis of hydrocephalus can be reached, and the diagnostic tools that may be beneficial can vary depending on the age of the patient and the underlying cause of the hydrocephalus. In instances of hydrocephalus secondary to an intracranial tumor, cross-sectional imaging is the most effective diagnostic modality for identifying the location and severity of the inciting tumor, as well as the severity of the hydrocephalus. Both computed tomography (CT) and MRI can be useful in making a diagnosis; however, MRI is superior for identifying and characterizing focal lesions, particularly those within the caudal fossa. MRI also allows for superior soft tissue detail that can help differentiate between an incidental normotensive

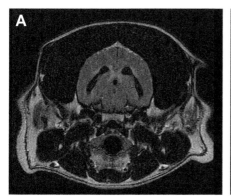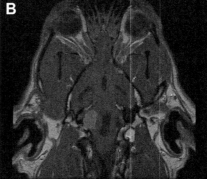

Fig. 1. Transverse T2 FLAIR magnetic resonance images at the level of the rostral colliculus (A) and dorsal T1-weighted postcontrast images of a dog with a mass arising within the right lateral metencephalon (B) resulting in expansion of the lateral, third, and fourth ventricles, and the mesencephalic aqueduct. Periventricular FLAIR hyperintensity can be noted on the transverse sequence.

chronic hydrocephalus, versus an acute hypertensive hydrocephalus.[8] This is an important distinction to make, as an incidental normotensive hydrocephalus should not be treated by way of a VP shunt, whereas shunt placement can be vital in managing acute neurologic decline in cases of acute obstructive hydrocephalus.

One of the most notable features that can distinguish an acute hydrocephalus from a chronic normotensive hydrocephalus is the presence of periventricular edema. On CT, this may appear as blurred ventricular margins and hypoattenuation of the periventricular parenchyma. On MRI, periventricular edema is often best seen on fluid-attenuated inversed recovery (FLAIR) sequences as periventricular FLAIR hyperintensity[8] (**Fig. 1**). Other MRI features that have been shown to differentiate clinical from nonclinical hydrocephalus include the elevation of the corpus callosum, dorsoventral flattening of the interthalamic adhesion, dilation of the olfactory recesses, thinning of the cortical sulci and/or the subarachnoid space, and disruption of the internal capsule adjacent to the caudate nucleus.[9] The ventricular distribution of hydrocephalus is typically upstream from the location of the obstruction (**Fig. 2**).

The decision to place a VP shunt should be made based on diagnostic imaging in conjunction with clinical signs. It is important to recognize that with acute obstructive hydrocephalus secondary to an intracranial tumor, the degree of hydrocephalus and the amount of cerebral cortical atrophy is likely much less significant than is typically seen in patients with congenital hydrocephalus. Neurologic signs may be severe despite a subjectively mild enlargement of the ventricles. Other imaging findings, such as periventricular hyperintensity, can help support an obstructive hydrocephalus as the cause of clinical decline even when only mild changes are present.

While MRI may be the best modality for making an initial diagnosis, CT becomes a crucial tool when it comes to surgical planning. Once an acute obstructive hydrocephalus has been identified, CT should be used for planning burr hole location, catheter angle, and depth of the ventricular catheter. This is a particularly important step, as there is often a much smaller target area in which to place the catheter due to a usually thicker brain parenchyma and smaller ventricles when compared to chronic congenital cases. If there is lateral ventricular asymmetry, the general rule is to place the shunt so that the catheter resides within the larger ventricle. In some instances, bilateral catheterization is required if both lateral ventricles are affected and there is no communication between the two. In this situation, placing a single shunt may relieve the

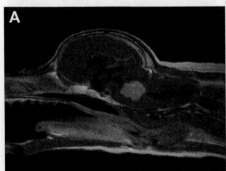
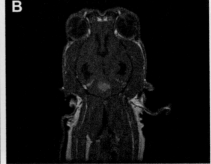

Fig. 2. Midline sagittal (*A*) and dorsal (*B*) T1-weighted postcontrast MR images of a dog with a suspected choroid plexus tumor of the fourth ventricle. There is visible enlargement of the lateral ventricles, third ventricle, and the mesencephalic aqueduct secondary to downstream obstruction of CSF flow.

pressure in one hemisphere of the brain; however, a hypertensive hydrocephalus could still be present or later develop within the other hemisphere necessitating a second surgery.

EQUIPMENT AND MATERIALS

A number of commercially available VP shunt systems are available. All of these systems contain the same basic components, which include a fenestrated proximal ventricular catheter, a valve system, and distal tubing. There is some variation in the valve configuration and additives to the tubing. Different valve mechanisms include slit valves, diaphragm valves, adjustable valves, and ruby ball valves. Systems may include prechambers, Rickham reservoirs, and antisiphon mechanisms that can alter the location of the valve relative to the catheter to facilitate ease of placement in different patients. While adjustable flow valves may be associated with a lower complication rate in humans, they are generally cost-prohibitive in companion animals.

The authors have a preference for the Codman–Hakim fixed pressure valve system (70–120 mm H$_2$O) with an inline Rickham reservoir or a prechamber depending on the shape or configuration of the VP shunt (**Fig. 3**). Valves can come in low-pressure, medium-pressure, and high-pressure systems. While opinions differ as to which pressure valve is best, the authors prefer the medium fixed pressure as it more closely resembles normal ICP in dogs (7.2 $\pm$ 2.3 mm Hg).[10] In addition to this, the Hakim valve system utilizes a small, synthetic ruby ball to control the flow of CSF. The smooth surface of this valve is designed to make it less susceptible to proteinaceous buildup, which decreases the risk of obstruction.[11]

Prechambers and Rickham reservoirs allow for greater manipulation of flow through the system, as they can be used for drawing CSF for analysis, flushing of the system, and to help troubleshoot should issues arise. There are various configurations and sizes of this valve and catheter system that can be selected based on patient size and surgeon preference. The authors prefer a "nonunitized" variant for brain tumors with highly proteinaceous CSF to help facilitate valve replacement in the event of complications in the future. This variant is also a reasonable choice in patients with brain tumors underlying their hydrocephalus as they are typically not still growing, unlike most patients with congenital hydrocephalus secondary to developmental abnormalities.

IMPLANTATION OF THE VENTRICULOPERITONEAL SHUNT

Placement of a VP shunt has a relatively high failure rate, making thorough planning and execution essential. It is strongly recommended to use recent preoperative

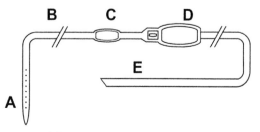

Fig. 3. A ventriculoperitoneal shunt system with a prechamber. (A) Ventricular catheter. (B) Proximal shunt tubing. (C) Prechamber. (D) Valve system. (E) Distal tubing. (Dr Katharine Russell, MVB.)

imaging for surgical planning. This allows for more accurate planning of the required depth and angle of the ventricular catheter. This is particularly important in patients who may have abnormal intraventricular anatomy due to a brain tumor, which may change over time and with progression of hydrocephalus.

The proximal catheter of the shunt is inserted into the lateral ventricle through a small burr hole within the skull. The one-way valve and reservoir are typically anchored dorsal to the ipsilateral ear near the base of the skull. The distal catheter is passed

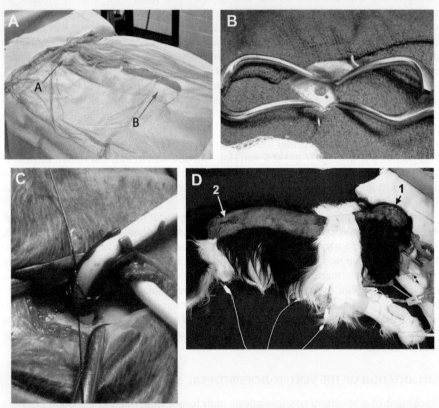

Fig. 4. (*A*) Positioning and draping of a patient in preparation for a VP shunt. The surgical field includes the area of the skull where the ventricular catheter will be inserted (A), the lateral abdomen where the distal tubing will enter the peritoneal cavity (B), and the lateral neck and body wall along which the distal tubing will be passed. (*B*) A burr hole is drilled within the skull at desired shunt location. A smaller anchoring hole is drilled adjacent to the burr hole, which is used for anchoring the right-angle connector to the skull. (*C*) Anchoring of the right-angle connector with nylon suture using a finger trap pattern. (*D*) Immediate postoperative view of a patient following VP shunt placement showing the location of the cranial incision for the ventricular portion (1) and the abdominal incision for the distal portion (2). Note that the patient is shaved along the length of the path of the shunt. (*From* [*A–C*] Thomas W, Narak J. Shunt Placement and Marsupialization in Treatment of Hydrocephalus and Quadrigeminal Diverticula. In: Shores A, Brisson BA, editors. Current techniques in canine and feline neurosurgery. John Wiley & Sons; 2017 with permission. [*D*] Thomas WB. Hydrocephalus in dogs and cats. Vet Clin North Am Small Anim Pract. 2010;40(1):143–159.)

subcutaneously along the lateral neck and chest wall, with the end passed into the peritoneal cavity via a flank incision. The peritoneal cavity is the most common location of termination and is associated with the least complications in human literature; however, alternative termination sites have been used in humans, including the pleural space, right atrium, or gallbladder, but these locations are typically reserved for situations where insertion into the peritoneal cavity is contraindicated.[12]

The patient should be positioned in lateral recumbency, with the head at approximately a 45° angle relative to the body. Towels, sandbags, or a vacuum-assisted positioning system should be used to secure the head in place in a slightly elevated position. The patient's skin should be clipped and surgically prepared over the entirety of the dorsal skull, along the entire subcutaneous route of the lateral neck and chest, and past the abdominal entry point of the distal catheter (**Fig. 4**A). A curvilinear incision is made adjacent to the sagittal crest, and the temporalis muscle is incised at the origins and reflected ventrally. At the desired location, a burr hole is created that is slightly larger than the catheter. A smaller hole immediately caudal to this hole is also created to facilitate securing the catheter in place (**Fig. 4**B).

Prior to opening the dura, a small incision is made in the flank approximately 3 to 4 cm caudal to the last rib to facilitate blunt dissection into the abdominal cavity. Dissection should be made through the external abdominal oblique, internal abdominal oblique, and transversus abdominis muscles in the direction of the muscle fibers. A shunt passer or Doyen forceps is then passed subcutaneously from the cranial incision caudally to the abdominal incision. In larger dogs, an additional incision along the tunnel may be necessary to help facilitate this. The distal portion of the shunt is typically pulled or tunneled alongside the passer. Care should be taken to angle the distal end of the passer away from the chest wall so as not to accidentally puncture the chest wall. Ideally, the passer is inserted through a small window under the muscle at the base of the skull, which allows the catheter to sit flush against the skull and allows for better anchoring of the shunt. Alternatively, the passer can be inserted from caudal to cranial, and the distal catheter, whether unitized or nonunitized, can then be pulled back through the subcutaneous space using the passer. The distal end of the catheter should be placed on a sterile surface while proceeding with the placement of the ventricular portion.

Once the shunt has tunneled into place, a small nick in the dura is made using a 25 gauge needle or scalpel. The ventricular catheter is then inserted to premeasured depth. A CSF sample should be obtained at this time. Ensure to clamp off the catheter during this process to avoid overdrainage of the ventricle. The proximal catheter should then be attached to the valve, completing the system. The proximal catheter and valve should be secured in place with a finger-trap made from nonabsorbable suture and anchored to the skull using the small hole drilled caudal to the burr hole earlier in the process (**Fig. 4**C). Take care to observe for CSF flow within the valve and out of the distal abdominal portion of the catheter prior to inserting the catheter into the abdomen to ensure the entirety of the system is patent. Cutting the distal end of the catheter is often necessary to optimize the length. Typically, 1.5 to 2 times the length of the abdomen is recommended for the length of the inserted portion. In some catheter types, it may be beneficial to fenestrate the distal tube to reduce the likelihood of blockage or obstruction by abdominal viscera or mesentery. The abdominal wall incision is closed via a purse-string suture and routine skin closure. The cranial incision is closed routinely after ensuring that the ventricular catheter is secured[13] (**Fig. 4**D). Cross-sectional imaging is recommended postoperatively to ensure that the placement of the catheter is satisfactory.

ADVERSE EVENTS/CHALLENGES

There are 3 categories of complications that can be experienced following shunt placement. These categories include mechanical failures, functional failures, and infection. Mechanical failures are the most common cause for shunt failures in small animals.[14] This category of complications includes shunt obstruction, ventricular collapse due to overshunting, disconnection of the shunt components, or migration of the shunt. Uniquely challenging to VP shunts used in patients with brain tumors is the potential for tumor emboli or CSF with a high protein concentration to clog the shunt. A protein content of greater than 4 g/L (400 mg/dL) is reported to clog most VP shunt valves, though clogging can occur even with much lower protein content.[15] An additional complicating factor in shunt placement in dogs with acute obstructive hydrocephalus is that there is typically a smaller target area in which to place the shunt and an increased risk for blockage of the shunt catheter as the ventricular diameter recedes to normal. Many of these complications can be avoided through careful surgical planning and equipment selection, using sound surgical technique, and employing prophylactic antibiotics following surgery. However, even when all necessary care

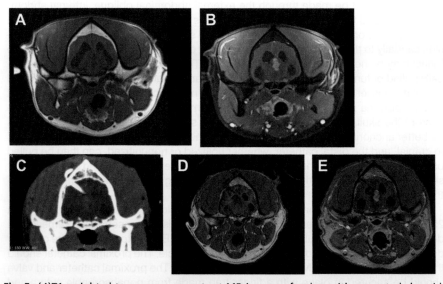

Fig. 5. (A)T1-weighted transverse precontrast MR images of a dog with suspected choroid plexus tumor of the third ventricle. There is bilateral enlargement of the lateral ventricles, which is slightly more pronounced on the right. (B) T1-weighted transverse postcontrast MR images of the same dog showing the strongly and uniformly contrast-enhancing mass within the third ventricle resulting in upstream ventriculomegaly. (C) Computed tomography of the same dog postventriculoperitoneal shunt placement. The ventricular catheter can be seen residing within the right lateral ventricle. A slight reduction in right lateral ventricular size can be appreciated. (D) T1-weighted transverse precontrast MRI of the same patient 1 month later, prior to radiation therapy. The ventricular catheter is in place, and a subtle reduction in the ventricular volume can be noted in this ventricle. (E) T1-weighted transverse postcontrast MRI of the same patient 1 month postradiation therapy. There is bilateral ventricular enlargement compared to the previous image indicating shunt obstruction. This patient had proteinaceous debris within the valve, necessitating a valve replacement.

is taken, some complications cannot be avoided and intervention including surgical revision may be necessary (**Fig. 5**).

TROUBLESHOOTING

As discussed, there is a relatively high complication rate in patients with an implanted VP shunt. It is imperative that the clinician is able to recognize, localize, and trouble-shoot when there is an apparent complication associated with the shunt. Typically, these patients present with an acute recurrence of clinical signs with forebrain localization.

Ideally, any patient known to have a VP shunt implanted who presents with these clinical signs should be reimaged. The first step is to perform survey radiography to ensure that none of the shunt components have disconnected. Once this has been determined, cross-sectional imaging, ideally an MRI, should be performed. MRI can determine the positioning of the ventricular catheter and assess for subdural hema-toma, ventricular collapse, periventricular edema, or further progression of hydro-cephalus. In some cases, there will be contralateral ventricular expansion if ventricular outflow is blocked, or there may be ipsilateral ventricular expansion if the issue is shunt related. Changes in tumor size or local metastases can also be detected at this stage.

Assessment of CSF flow can be determined, in some cases, percutaneously with gentle CSF aspiration of the Rickham reservoir or prechamber. This should be per-formed with extreme care and aseptic technique. A CSF sample can also be taken here to assess for infection. Open assessment can be performed in surgery and may facilitate more confidence in the detection of CSF flow through the system. Visual inspection of the valve to look for cellular debris, blood clots, and to determine whether flow is continuous should be performed. Gentle and minimal pumping with strategic occlusion of the proximal tubing, the tubing between the prechamber and the valve, and then the tubing distal to the valve can help identify where the occlusion has occurred. In addition, drawing from the reservoir and assessing the refill can deter-mine the patency of the ventricular catheter. Flow through the valve can be assessed by gentle flushing of saline through the system. Valvular occlusion can be remedied by gentle pumping and flushing. Care should be taken not to excessively pump or flush the system as it may cause overdrainage or damage the valve mechanism, respectively.

If the obstruction cannot be remedied, the valve or other affected component can be replaced if using a nonunitized variant of the system. The same meticulous attention to detail should be used when replacing shunt components. In some cases, with contra-lateral ventricular expansion, a shunt can be placed on that side.

In some tumors with excessive proteinaceous debris and repeated failure of VP shunt, a lateral ventriculostomy as described by Shores and colleagues[16] (**Fig. 6**) may be a viable salvage technique in managing these rare but challenging cases.

DISCUSSION

VP shunting is considered the standard of care for severe clinical obstructive hydro-cephalus. While the majority of literature regarding VP shunt placement pertains to treatment in younger patients with suspected congenital causes, the surgical proced-ure and complication profile are similar in patients with acquired hydrocephalus sec-ondary to brain tumors. However, patients with brain tumors present distinct challenges compared to those with congenital hydrocephalus. Patients with friable tu-mors or higher CSF protein content may have an increased risk for shunt valve

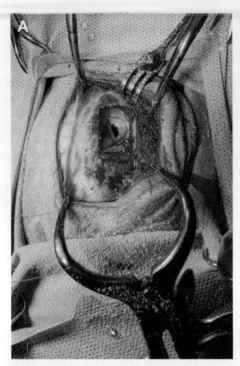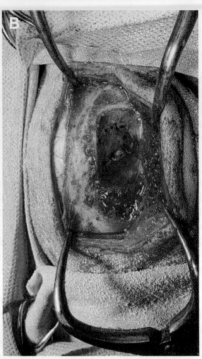

Fig. 6. Intraoperative images displaying sequences during a lateral ventriculostomy proced-ure. The left image (*A*) depicts the completed fenestration and eversion of the lateral ventricle. The right image (*B*) depicts the completed duroplasty with swine intestinal submu-cosa. (*Images courtesy* of Dr Andy Shores, DVM, MS, PhD, DACVIM (Neurology).)

obstruction. Additionally, radiation therapy may initially result in tumor necrosis, potentially leading to valve obstruction by tumor emboli. These risk factors are impor-tant to consider when selecting the type of shunt and how the shunt is placed. To miti-gate these risks and simplify revision when required, the authors recommend using a valve with a Rickham reservoir and a nonunitized catheter system. A nonunitized sys-tem allows for an easier valve replacement without the need to remove the entire cath-eter system when revision is required. Despite the inherent complications and challenges unique to patients with brain tumors, VP shunting can provide rapid, effec-tive, and durable relief from clinical signs of hydrocephalus secondary to brain tumors, especially when used in conjunction with other treatments such as radiation, chemo-therapy, or surgery. Patients with progressive clinical signs of obstructive hydroceph-alus are ideal candidates for VP shunting, with ventricular system neoplasms and tumors affecting the caudal fossa being the most common tumor types associated with acute hydrocephalus. Proper planning and execution of the VP shunting proced-ure are crucial to minimize complications that can include mechanical failures, func-tional failures, and infection. Recognizing obstructive hydrocephalus on MRI in patients with brain tumors may be more challenging compared to congenital cases. Nevertheless, VP shunting can help alleviate clinical signs attributable to hydroceph-alus and reduce risk in patients requiring multiple anesthesia events for treatment. VP shunting directly addresses the pathophysiologic changes caused by hydrocephalus, leading to rapid clinical improvement and reduced anesthetic risk. These benefits contribute to both an improved quality of life and increased survival time making VP shun placement a key intervention for managing obstructive hydrocephalus secondary to brain tumors.

SUMMARY

- Brain tumors can cause obstructive hydrocephalus, which is often the major driver of clinical signs, especially in tumors arising within the ventricular system.
- VP shunting can provide rapid, effective, and durable relief from clinical signs of hydrocephalus secondary to brain tumors when used alone; however, it is more effective alongside other treatments such as radiation, chemotherapy, or surgery.
- VP shunting may offer standalone benefits to survival in patients, even without radiation therapy or surgery.
- Patients with progressive clinical signs of obstructive hydrocephalus, particularly those with ventricular system neoplasms or tumors affecting the caudal fossa, are ideal candidates for VP shunting.
- Other MRI features associated with clinical hydrocephalus include elevation of the corpus callosum, dorsoventral flattening of the interthalamic adhesion, dilation of the olfactory recesses, thinning of the cortical sulci and/or the subarachnoid space, and disruption of the internal capsule adjacent to the caudate nucleus.
- Meticulous planning and execution of the VP shunting procedure are essential to minimizing complications, which can include mechanical failures, functional failures, and infection.
- An additional surgical challenge commonly experienced with VP shunt placement in patients with brain tumors is that there is a smaller target area in which to place the shunt.

CLINICS CARE POINTS

- VP shunting is considered the gold standard surgical intervention for managing obstructive hydrocephalus.
- VP shunting can provide rapid, effective, and durable relief from clinical signs of hydrocephalus secondary to brain tumors when used alone; however, it is more effective alongside other treatments such as radiation, chemotherapy, or surgery.
- Studies have found that VP shunting followed by radiation therapy resulted in a longer survival time than VP shunting or radiation therapy alone in patients with hydrocephalus secondary to neoplasia.
- Patients with progressive clinical signs of obstructive hydrocephalus, particularly those with ventricular system neoplasms or tumors affecting the caudal fossa, are ideal candidates for VP shunting.
- MRI is superior for identifying and characterizing focal lesions, while CT is crucial for surgical planning of VP shunt placement.
- Periventricular edema, seen as blurred ventricular margins on CT and periventricular FLAIR hyperintensity on MRI, can help distinguish acute hydrocephalus from chronic normotensive hydrocephalus or ventriculomegaly.
- Patients with acute obstructive hydrocephalus are less likely to experience ventricular collapse following VP shunt placement due to less parenchymal atrophy but are typically at greater risk for the obstruction of the shunt valve due to friable tumors or increased CSF protein content.

> • Using a valve with a Rickham reservoir or a prechamber and a nonunitized valve system can help mitigate the risks associated with shunt valve obstruction in patients with brain tumors and make troubleshooting easier.

DISCLOSURE

The authors declare that this chapter was written in the absence of any commercial or financial relationsips that could be construed as a potential conflict of interest.

REFERENCES

1. Westworth DR, Dickinson PJ, Vernau W, et al. Choroid plexus tumors in 56 dogs (1985-2007). J Vet Intern Med 2008;22(5):1157–65.
2. Thomas WB. Hydrocephalus in dogs and cats. Vet Clin North Am Small Anim Pract 2010;40(1):143–59.
3. Wisner ER, Dickinson PJ, Higgins RJ. Magnetic resonance imaging features of canine intracranial neoplasia. Vet Radiol Ultrasound 2011;52(1 Suppl 1):S52–61.
4. Schmidt M, Ondreka N. Hydrocephalus in Animals. In: Cinalli G, Özek M, Sainte-Rose C, editors. Pediatric hydrocephalus. Switzerland: Springer Nature; 2019. p. 53–95.
5. Troxel MT, Vite CH, Van Winkle TJ, et al. Feline intracranial neoplasia: retrospective review of 160 cases (1985-2001). J Vet Intern Med 2003;17(6):850–9.
6. Orlandi R, Vasilache CG, Mateo I. Palliative ventriculoperitoneal shunting in dogs with obstructive hydrocephalus caused by tumors affecting the third ventricle. J Vet Intern Med 2020;34(4):1556–62.
7. Beckmann K, Kowalska M, Meier V. Solitary intraventricular tumors in dogs and cats treated with radiotherapy alone or combined with ventriculoperitoneal shunts: A retrospective descriptive case series. J Vet Intern Med 2023;37(1): 204–15.
8. Przyborowska P, Adamiak Z, Jaskolska M, et al. Hydrocephalus in dogs: a review. Vet Med-Czech 2013;58(2):73–80.
9. Laubner S, Ondreka N, Failing K, et al. Magnetic resonance imaging signs of high intraventricular pressure–comparison of findings in dogs with clinically relevant internal hydrocephalus and asymptomatic dogs with ventriculomegaly. BMC Vet Res 2015;11:181.
10. Sturges BK, Dickinson PJ, Tripp LD, et al. Intracranial pressure monitoring in normal dogs using subdural and intraparenchymal miniature strain-gauge transducers. J Vet Intern Med 2019;33(2):708–16.
11. Filgueiras Rda R, Martins Cde S, de Almeida RM, et al. Long-term evaluation of a new ventriculoperitoneal shunt valve system in a dog. J Vet Emerg Crit Care 2009;19(6):623–8.
12. Lee P, DiPatri AJ. Evaluation of suspected cerebrospinal fluid shunt complications in children. Clin Pediatr Emerg Med 2008;9(2):76–82.
13. Thomas W, Narak J. Shunt Placement and Marsupialization in Treatment of Hydrocephalus and Quadrigeminal Diverticula. In: Shores A, Brisson BA, editors. Current techniques in canine and feline neurosurgery. Hoboken NJ: John Wiley & Sons; 2017. p. 129–37.
14. Gradner G, Kaefinger R, Dupré G. Complications associated with ventriculoperitoneal shunts in dogs and cats with idiopathic hydrocephalus: A systematic review. J Vet Intern Med 2019;33(2):403–12.

15. Pople IK. Hydrocephalus and shunts: what the neurologist should know. J Neurol Neurosurg Psychiatry 2002;73(Suppl 1):i17–22.
16. Shores A, Kornberg S, Beasley MB, et al. Fenestration of the lateral ventricle in management of obstructive hydrocephalus in young small animals. In: Proceedings of the American college of Veterinary internal Medicine Forum 2015. Lakewood CO: American College of Veterinary Internal Medicine; 2015. Available at: http://www.vin.com/acvim/2015/default.htm.

Intraoperative Ultrasound in Brain Surgery

Alison M. Lee, DVM, MS, DACVR,
Andy Shores, DVM, MS, PhD, DACVIM (Neurology)*

KEYWORDS

- Intraoperative ultrasound • Intracranial surgery • Brain tumors • Probe selection

KEY POINTS

- Real-time imaging provides the neurosurgeon guidance in resection of intracranial masses.
- Doppler imaging helps to identify surrounding vasculature.
- Borders between the mass and normal cortical tissue/vital structures can be identified.
- The completeness of resection of the mass can be evaluated intraoperatively using this technique.

 Video content accompanies this article at http://www.vetsmall.theclinics.com.

INTRODUCTION

When possible, maximal and safe surgical resection of intracranial tumors optimizes the therapeutic protocols. Intraoperative ultrasound (IOUS) is becoming increasingly utilized in veterinary neurosurgery and continued advancement of this discipline requires accurate real-time localization and visualization of the mass.[1] In the human neurosurgical realm, within the last decade, intraoperative MRI and intraoperative computed tomography (CT) have been employed as a means of intraoperative imaging; however, these tools are not true real-time imaging modalities and are also often less accurate in differentiating borders between normal tissue and tumor than IOUS.[2] In addition, intraoperative CT and MRI are likely well beyond the financial reach of the veterinary neurosurgeon. A description of the utility if IOUS for veterinary neurosurgery was first presented in 2012[3] and additional information was published in 2021.[4]

Department of Clinical Science, College of Veterinary Medicine, Mississippi State Univeristy, 240 Wise Center Drive, Mississippi State, MS 39762, USA
* Corresponding author.
E-mail address: shores@cvm.msstate.edu

Vet Clin Small Anim 55 (2025) 149–155
https://doi.org/10.1016/j.cvsm.2024.07.012   vetsmall.theclinics.com

ADVANTAGES AND DISADVANTAGES OF INTRAOPERATIVE ULTRASOUND

The obvious advantages of this technique are real-time visualization of the intracranial mass, surrounding vasculature using the Doppler mode, visualization of surrounding structures (ventricles, important anatomic structures), and distinguishing the borders between mass and normal cortical tissue. IOUS is accurate even in the face of any brain-shift and is considered the only real-time imaging modality for intracranial surgeries. The disadvantage is the cost of the equipment and the learning curve needed to use IOUS to its full advantage.[2] Ultrasound equipment is standard in all specialty practices, so just a few things need consideration in preparing to utilize this modality in the operating room.

TECHNIQUE AND PRODUCING QUALITY IMAGES

In adult and larger juvenile patients, calvarial bone will generally limit brain sonography, as ultrasound cannot penetrate the bone. Therefore, IOUS is performed either by imaging through a pre-existing break in the calvarial bone or via the surgical calvarial osteotomy.

Probes are cleaned and are placed inside sterile sleeves, along with sterile coupling gel (**Fig. 1**). The sleeve is secured to the surgical field. Air bubbles trapped within the sleeve can result in artifacts while scanning, so keeping the sleeve tight over the probe head is recommended. Probe/patient contact is maintained by a combination of sterile ultrasound gel within the sterile sleeve and infusion of sterile saline into the surgical site.

Scanning is accomplished via a combination of sweeping/sliding (translation of the probe across the surgical field) and fanning/rocking (tilting the probe without translational movement to change the angle of insonation) of the probe within the surgical field in both the transverse and sagittal planes. Translational movement of the probe is usually limited by the size of the craniotomy; thus, the majority of IOUS is accomplished via fanning and rocking while the probe remains in the same location.

Generally, sweeping motions at the start of the scan can assist in identifying anatomic landmarks within the surgical field. These can be compared to pre-surgical MRI or CT imaging for confirmation. Once a lesion is identified, margins and lesion depth can be measured via the electronic calipers. Color Doppler should

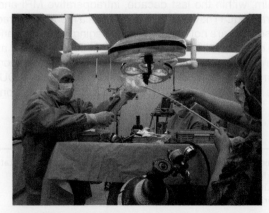

Fig. 1. The ultrasound probe has been cleaned and is being passed to the surgeon, placing it in a sterile, plastic sleeve that contains sterile coupling gel. After the probe has been secured on the sterile field, it is ready to be used to image the brain through the craniotomy site.

be used to locate any vessels both within the lesion and within the surrounding surgical field prior to any surgical intervention. It is important to note the potential for significant shifting of anatomy during surgery because of both manipulation and removal of tissue and the introduction of saline and hemorrhage into the site; thus, it may be necessary to reorient to more static anatomy multiple times during the examination period. IOUS is also used to facilitate placement of biopsy equipment or other surgical instruments, as well as to identify the origination of any hemorrhage that occurs intraoperatively.

PROBE SELECTION

Probe selection (**Fig. 2**) is crucial for successful intraoperative sonography. For most small animal patients, a linear or microconvex probe, ranging from 7.5 to 12 mHz, will provide the best image quality.[1] These probes are often identical to those used in abdominal scanning. Although linear probes can be successfully employed while scanning the brain parenchyma, microconvex probes are generally superior due to the geometry of the probe head. Microconvex probes have a curved array, which most often fits better into the window created by the calvarial ostectomy. This geometry not only produces a higher quality scan, but it also limits the inclusion of gas bubbles from infused saline into the field of view, which can cause artifact in the underlying anatomy.

CASE EXAMPLES
Case 1

An 8 year old spayed female domestic long-haired cat was presented for a 6 month history of occasional complex-partial motor seizures. She had been on a course of antibiotics and received 2 doses of dexamethasone prior to referral. The neurologic examination was normal; however, the cat acted painful on palpation around the head and neck area. An MRI revealed a large, extra-axial, multilobular, T1 and T2 iso-to hyperintense, heterogeneously contrast enhancing mass along midline dorsally (**Fig. 3**). A right, rostrotentorial craniectomy was performed and the full extent of the mass was identified using IOUS, displaying a clear border between cortical tissue and mass. The IOUS was also beneficial in identifying residual portions of the tumor

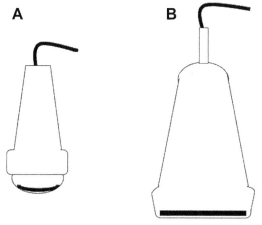

A   **B**

Fig. 2. The 2 types of recommended ultrasound probes for intracranial imaging: (*A*) microconvex probe and (*B*) linear probe.

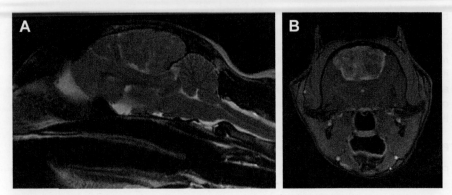

Fig. 3. MRI of a large, extra-axial, multilobular, T1 and T2 iso-to hyperintense, heterogeneously contrast enhancing mass along midline dorsally. (*A*) Sagittal T2-weighted image; (*B*) transverse T1-weighted image with contrast.

as the surgery progressed and there was considerable brain-shift (**Fig. 4**). Microscopic evaluation of the mass identified it as a meningioma, transitional type.

Case 2

An 11 year old male, neutered Boston Terrier was presented for evaluation of a 1 month history of generalized motor seizures. An MRI performed at a referral practice revealed a large, intra-axial, T1 isointense and T2 hyperintense, fluid-filled mass in the right piriform lobe (**Fig. 5**A, B). Surgery consisted of a right, rostrotentorial craniectomy, identification of the mass via IOUS (**Fig. 5**C, Video 1), biopsy of the mass, and total gross resection of the mass using a Cavitron Ultrasonic Surgical Aspirator device (ªIntega Life Sciences). The histopathology revealed a high-grade astrocytoma.

Case 3

A 10 year old neutered male Boxer was presented for a 3 week history of seizures. An MRI revealed a large, intra-axial, T1 isointense and T2 hyperintense, fluid-filled mass in the right parietal lobe (**Fig. 6**A–C). A right, rostrotentorial Craniectomy was performed, and the identification and the removal of the mass were similar as described in case 2.

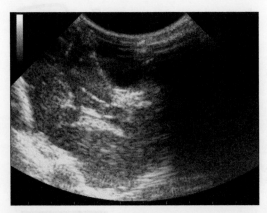

Fig. 4. Intraoperative ultrasound image of the brain in a sagittal orientation during tumor removal in Case 1. The mass is hyperechoic and sits deep to an anechoic pocket of fluid representing the portion of the mass already removed.

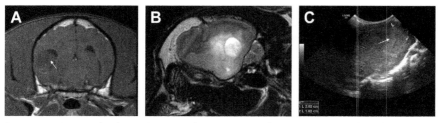

Fig. 5. An MRI reveals a large, intra-axial, T1 isointense (*A*, transverse view) and T2 hyperintense (*B*, sagittal view), fluid-filled mass in the right piriform lobe (*arrow*). Intraoperative ultrasound image of the brain in a sagittal orientation (*C*) shows the mass (*arrow*) as a smoothly marginated, hyperechogenic structure measuring 2.02 cm by 1.62 cm.

The IOUS images are seen in **Fig. 6**D, E, and exactly matched the measurements seen on the MRI. In 6E, a biopsy probe (arrow) is seen in the image and is being guided by the ultrasound. The mass was identified as a high-grade oligodendriglioma.

Case 4

A 9 year old female, spayed Schnauzer presented with a 2 year history of generalized motor seizures that had become more frequent and more severe despite continued anti-epileptic medications (phenobarbital). An MRI revealed a contrast enhancing mass in the left frontal lobe and adjacent to the falx-cerebri (**Fig. 7**A, B). A transfrontal

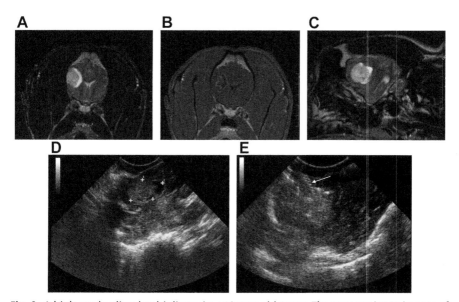

Fig. 6. A high-grade oligodendriglioma in a 10 year old Boxer. The top row is MR images of a large, intra-axial, T1 isointense and T2 hyperintense, fluid-filled mass in the right parietal lobe ((*A*) T2-weighted transverse image; (*B*) T1-weighted transverse image; (*C*) T2-weighted sagittal image). Below are 2 IOUS images. (*D*) The brain in a sagittal orientation and the mass as a smoothly marginated, iso-to hyperechoic structure measuring 2.20 cm by 1.32 cm. which is surrounded by anechoic fluid. (*E*) The insertion of a catheter into the lesion (*arrow*).

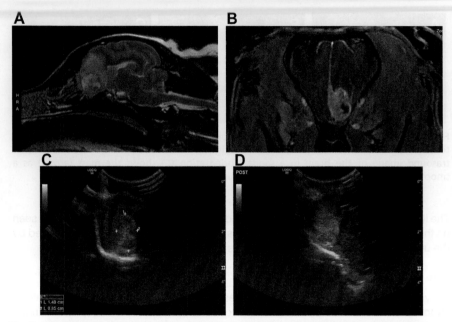

Fig. 7. The MRI revealed a large, extra-axial, strongly contrast enhancing mass rostrally on the left. (*A*) Sagittal T2-weighted image. (*B*) Transverse T1-weighted image with contrast. (*C, D*) Intra-operative ultrasound images of the brain in a sagittal orientation and show the mass as a smoothly marginated, hyperechoic structure measuring 1.49 cm by 0.85 cm. (*D*) The change in shape of the mass after IOUS-guided biopsy.

craniotomy was performed. Intraoperative identification of the mass was made using IOUS (**Fig. 7**C, D) and initially a biopsy was performed using the IOUS to guide the biopsy probe.

DISCUSSION

In our experience, IOUS has proven an invaluable addition to intracranial surgery, especially in real-time localization of the mass, identifying borders between mass and normal cerebral tissue, and identifying vascular supply to the mass. Our findings over the past several years agree with a human neurosurgery paper that states glial tumors appear hyperechogenic, often with areas of irregularity and the presence of central necrosis, cystic area, or hemorrhage. Meningiomas appear more uniformly hyperechogenic and have the clearest borders.[5] The future of IOUS is already making inroads into the discipline in human neurosurgery and includes contrast ultrasound techniques, elastography to differentiate normal tissue from tumor, and fusion techniques that pair real time B-scan ultrasound with other forms of cross-sectional imaging (MRI, CT, PET scans).[2] The authors are confident that continued work with IOUS will generate continued and expanded interest in this modality and continued reports of IOUS will foster its continued advancement.

SUMMARY

This study describes the essential components and the technique of IOUS. Case examples are given to illustrate the value and the accuracy of IOUS in intracranial surgery of companion animals.

CLINICS CARE POINT

- Accurate intraoperative imaging is a valuable tool in managment / surgical removal of intracranial masses.

DISCLOSURE

The authors have nothing to disclose.

SUPPLEMENTARY DATA

Supplementary data to this article can be found online at https://doi.org/10.1016/j.cvsm.2024.07.012.

REFERENCES

1. Lee AM, Tollefson C, Shores A. Intraoperative ultrasound in intracranial surgery. In: Shores A, Brisson B, editors. Advanced techniques in canine and feline neurosurgery. Hoboken, NJ: John Wiley and Sons; 2023. p. 171–8.
2. Dixon L, Lim A, Grech-Sollars M, et al. Intraoperative ultrasound in brain tumor surgery: A review and implementation guide. Neurosurg Rev 2022;45(4):2503–15. Epub 2022 Mar 30. PMID: 35353266; PMCID: PMC9349149.
3. Shores A, Brinkman E, Beasley M, et al. Intraoperative ultrasound for intracranial surgery. Denver CO: Proced ACVIM Forum; 2012.
4. Shores A, Lee AM, Kornberg ST, et al. Intraoperative ultrasound applications in intracranial surgery. Front Vet Sci 2021;8:725867. PMID: 34869713; PMCID: PMC8635011.
5. Giammalva GR, Ferini G, Musso S, et al. Intraoperative ultrasound: emerging technology and novel applications in brain tumor surgery. Front Oncol 2022;12:818446. PMID: 35178348; PMCID: PMC8844995.

Moving?

Make sure your subscription moves with you!

To notify us of your new address, find your **Clinics Account Number** (located on your mailing label above your name), and contact customer service at:

Email: journalscustomerservice-usa@elsevier.com

800-654-2452 (subscribers in the U.S. & Canada)
314-447-8871 (subscribers outside of the U.S. & Canada)

Fax number: 314-447-8029

Elsevier Health Sciences Division
Subscription Customer Service
3251 Riverport Lane
Maryland Heights, MO 63043

*To ensure uninterrupted delivery of your subscription, please notify us at least 4 weeks in advance of move.

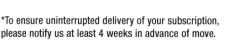

Moving?

Printed and bound by CPI Group (UK) Ltd, Croydon, CR0 4YY

08/05/2025

01864752-0007